María Teresa Hernández-Domínguez
María Plaza-Carmona

Prevention of hypothalamic amenorrhea in female athletes

María Teresa Hernández-Domínguez
María Plaza-Carmona

Prevention of hypothalamic amenorrhea in female athletes

Nutritional Guidelines

ScienciaScripts

Imprint
Any brand names and product names mentioned in this book are subject to trademark, brand or patent protection and are trademarks or registered trademarks of their respective holders. The use of brand names, product names, common names, trade names, product descriptions etc. even without a particular marking in this work is in no way to be construed to mean that such names may be regarded as unrestricted in respect of trademark and brand protection legislation and could thus be used by anyone.

Cover image: www.ingimage.com

This book is a translation from the original published under ISBN 978-620-0-02443-5.

Publisher:
Sciencia Scripts
is a trademark of
Dodo Books Indian Ocean Ltd. and OmniScriptum S.R.L publishing group

120 High Road, East Finchley, London, N2 9ED, United Kingdom
Str. Armeneasca 28/1, office 1, Chisinau MD-2012, Republic of Moldova, Europe
Managing Directors: Ieva Konstantinova, Victoria Ursu
info@omniscriptum.com

Printed at: see last page
ISBN: 978-620-8-62349-4

PREVENTION OF HYPOTHALAMIC AMENORRHOEA IN FEMALE ATHLETES

NUTRITIONAL GUIDELINES

MARÍA TERESA HERNÁNDEZ-DOMÍNGUEZ

MARIA PLAZA-CARMONA

INDEX

SUMMARY 3

1.INTRODUCTION 4

2.OBJECTIVES..12

3.METHODOLOGY 14

4.RESULTS..17

5.DISCUSSION...58

6.APPLICABILITY AND NEW LINES OF

RESEARCH..64

7.CONCLUSIONS 67

8.BIBLIOGRAPHY...69

SUMMARY

During normal puberty, the hypothalamus releases Gonadotropin Releasing Hormone (GnRH) in a pulsatile manner, and stimulates both the synthesis and secretion of Luteinising Hormone (LH) and Follicle Stimulating Hormone (FSH) from the anterior pituitary. Scientific literature has shown that in women with FHA (Functional Hypothalamic Amenorrhoea) GnRH secretion is suppressed, LH pulsatility is altered and total LH and FSH levels are reduced. As a consequence, there will be attenuated ovarian production of oestradiol, progesterone and testosterone, as well as subsequent anovulation and amenorrhoea. This suppression of the Hypothalamic-Pituitary-Ovarian Axis can be triggered by psychological stress, Eating Disorders (ED), weight loss and excessive exercise.Given that excessive exercise has been linked to the development of AHF especially in aesthetic sports and those in which weight plays a fundamental role such as athletics, sports nutrition, as well as the role of the sports nutritionist, will be fundamental pillars in both the prevention and treatment of this problem. The aim of this literature review was to gather relevant information on the mechanisms that trigger this pathology, as well as to focus on the nutritional guidelines that could prevent it. The diagnosis of Functional Hypothalamic Amenorrhea (FHA) due to low energy availability is a diagnosis by exclusion, after ruling out possible disorders that cause the absence of menstruation, such as Hypothyroidism, Hyperprolactinaemia, Polycystic Ovary Syndrome (PCOS), Ovarian Insufficiency and other pathologies. This often leads to an erroneous diagnosis of PCOS, which leads many women to follow nutritional guidelines that are not at all beneficial for the recovery of their menstrual cycle and their health.

Key words *Revision, Amenorrhoea Hypothalamic, Women Athletes, Energy Deficiency, Nutritional Therapy.*

1. INTRODUCTION

The percentage of women playing sport at all levels has increased dramatically over the last 50 years, as can be seen in the growing proportion of female Olympic athletes. At the Summer Olympics in Munich (1972), 15% of the participants were women, compared to 44% in London in 2012, the first Games in which women competed in all disciplines [(7)]. If we look at the last few Olympics it looks like the International Olympic Committee (IOC) has been promoting gender equality, and at the Tokyo 2020 Olympics, near equality was achieved with 48.8% female participation. The Paris 2024 Games are expected to continue this trend, with a goal of 50% female representation.

However, similar to the increasing participation of women in sport, elite female athletes are at a higher risk of suffering from a variety of injuries, including, most notably:

- Anterior Cruciate Ligament (ACL) injuries:

Women have a significantly higher incidence of ACL injuries than men, particularly in sports involving rapid changes of direction, jumping and landing, such as football, basketball and volleyball. Factors such as greater ligament laxity, differences in knee anatomy and movement patterns may contribute to this higher incidence.

- Iliotibial Cintilla Syndrome:

This syndrome, which causes pain in the lateral aspect of the knee, is more common in female runners and cyclists. The biomechanics and structure of the female pelvis may contribute to a greater predisposition to this injury.

- Stress Injuries (Stress Fractures):

Women are more prone to stress fractures, especially in endurance sports such as running and gymnastics. Risk factors include the female athlete's triad (eating disorder, amenorrhoea and osteoporosis), lower bone density and intensive training patterns.

- Tendinopathies:

Tendinopathies, such as patellar tendinitis (jumper's knee) and Achilles tendinitis, are common in women due to biomechanical and hormonal factors. Hormonal fluctuations throughout the menstrual cycle can affect the structure and function of collagen in tendons.

- Hip and pelvic problems:

Women have a different pelvic anatomy, which may contribute to a higher incidence of hip and pelvic injuries, such as iliotibial band friction syndrome, bursitis and acetabular labral injuries.

All of this is a consequence of different factors such as:

- Anatomy:

Women tend to have a wider pelvis and a greater Q-angle (angle formed by the hip line and knee line), which can influence the alignment and biomechanics of the lower limbs.

- Hormones:

Hormonal fluctuations, especially in oestrogen and relaxin, can affect joint stability and soft tissue strength, increasing the risk of injury.

- Biomechanics and Technique:

Differences in biomechanics and movement technique can influence the incidence of injury. Women tend to have different jumping, landing and running patterns compared to men.

- Psychosocial factors:

Social expectations and pressures to achieve certain standards of performance or appearance can influence training and nutrition habits, contributing to an increased risk of injury.

In this sense, we are going to focus the object of study of our work on stress fractures or endocrine disorders such as Functional Hypothalamic Amenorrhoea (FHA).

AHF is defined as the absence of menstruation caused by a suppression of the hypothalamic-pituitary-ovarian axis, for which no anatomical or organic cause can be found. It is potentially reversible and is often seen in situations of stress, weight loss or excessive exercise [1,7]. It is caused by a dysfunction of the hypothalamus, a region of the brain that regulates numerous bodily functions, including the menstrual cycle. This condition is not related to structural or anatomical diseases of the reproductive organs, but is functional, meaning that it is caused by external factors affecting the function of the hypothalamus.

Chronic stress, both physical (such as excessive exercise) and psychological (such as anxiety and depression), can alter the production of hormones necessary for ovulation and the menstrual cycle [1,7]. On the other hand, Low Body Weight and Eating Disorders are largely triggers. Low body mass index (BMI) and conditions such as anorexia nervosa can decrease the production of leptin, a hormone that regulates energy and appetite, negatively affecting hypothalamic function. Finally, note how physical exercise shows a high correlation with their development. It has been observed that high-performance athletes and people who engage in intense physical exercise may experience AHF due to decreased body fat and increased physical stress [1,7]. Physiologically it can manifest as primary or secondary amenorrhoea [1]. Primary amenorrhoea is defined as the absence of menarche at age 16 years with normal growth and development of secondary sexual characteristics, or, at age 14 years with absence of secondary sexual characteristics. Secondary amenorrhoea is defined as the absence of menstruation for more than three cycles in a row in a person who previously menstruated regularly, or more than six months in a woman with irregular cycles. FHA is the most common form of primary amenorrhoea in adolescents, while the most common form of its secondary variant is polycystic ovary syndrome (PCOS) and pregnancy [1]. The prevalence of amenorrhoea not due to pregnancy is approximately 3-4% [5].

- **Endocrine disruption associated with AHF**

During normal puberty, the hypothalamus releases Gonadotropin Releasing Hormone (GnRH) in a pulsatile manner, stimulating both the synthesis and secretion of Luteinising Hormone (LH) and Follicle Stimulating Hormone (FSH) from the anterior pituitary. This process is essential for normal reproductive development and function [1]. GnRH regulates the menstrual cycle by controlling the release of LH and FSH, which in turn promote follicular growth in the ovaries and the production of oestrogen and progesterone. However, scientific literature has shown that in women with Functional Hypothalamic Amenorrhoea (FHA), GnRH secretion is suppressed. This results in an impaired LH pulsatility and a reduction total LH and FSH levels [1,2]. This hormonal dysfunction results in attenuated ovarian production of oestradiol, progesterone and testosterone, leading to anovulation (lack of ovulation) and amenorrhoea (absence of menstruation). The decrease in these sex hormones can severely affect women's reproductive and general health, including bone density and cardiovascular health [1, 6,13)].

In addition, there is an induced activation of the hypothalamic-pituitary-adrenal axis, with a consequent increase in hypothalamic secretion of Corticotropin Releasing Hormone (CRH) and cortisol in the adrenal glands. The increase in cortisol, a stress hormone, together with endorphins released in response to intense physical activity, contributes to the inhibition of GnRH secretion by the hypothalamus. This negative feedback mechanism further exacerbates reproductive axis dysfunction, perpetuating gonadotropin suppression and maintaining amenorrhoea. The combination of physical and psychological stressors, together with hormonal disturbances, creates a physiological environment that inhibits normal reproductive function and can have long-term effects on female health (Figure 1).

In addition, Functional Hypothalamic Amenorrhoea (FHA) is associated with a hypometabolic state reflected by low levels of insulin and Insulin-like Growth Factor (IGF-I) and high levels of growth hormone and IGF-I binding protein. Because IGF-I stimulates the release of both GnRH and LH, a reduction in IGF-I activity may explain the reduction in LH secretion. In addition, serum levels of leptin, a marker of nutritional status also involved in pulsatile GnRH secretion, are markedly reduced in amenorrhoeic athletes, in addition to thyroxine and triiodothyronine levels. This indicates an altered metabolic state that negatively impacts reproductive function. Leptin, secreted by adipocytes, plays a crucial role in the regulation of energy homeostasis and reproductive function. Low leptin levels, as a result of low energy availability, can inhibit hypothalamic function and thus GnRH secretion.

Figure 1: Summary of endocrine disruptions associated athletic amenorrhoea [7].

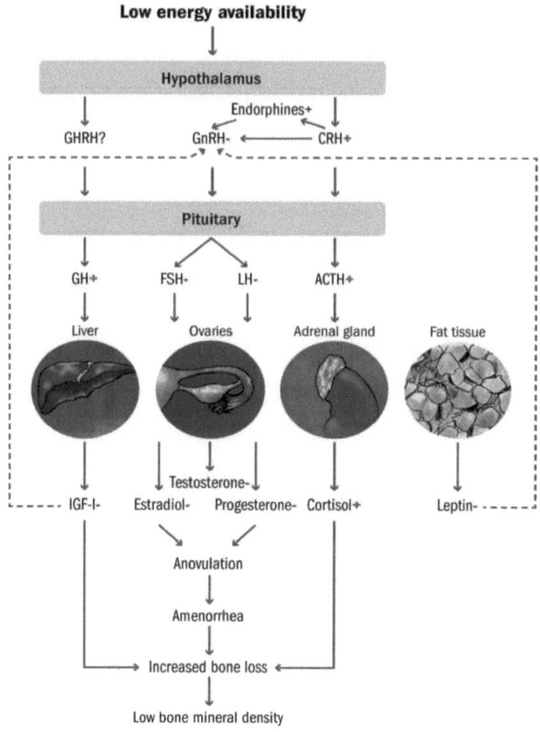

This hypometabolic state is also reflected in thyroid function, with reduced levels of thyroxine (T4) and triiodothyronine (T3), hormones essential for energy metabolism and overall body function. The reduction in these hormones can lead to symptoms of hypothyroidism, such as fatigue, cold intolerance and weight gain, further complicating the situation for athletes with AHF. In addition, elevated levels of growth hormone and IGF-I binding protein may be an adaptive response of the body to conserve energy in a state of prolonged calorie deficit. The interplay between these hormonal and metabolic factors creates an environment in which reproductive function is compromised as an energy-sparing strategy [7].Taken together, these findings indicate that AHF is due to central inhibition of the reproductive axis by stress hormones and endorphins, in combination with attenuated GnRH stimulation as a result of low levels of IGF-I and leptin. Leptin is a key hormone in energy homeostasis, secreted by adipocytes (adipose tissue cells) and regulates various functions through receptors on neurons in the hypothalamus [7]. Although leptin is secreted in proportion to body fat content, its levels vary dramatically in response to fasting, dietary restriction and overeating, even before significant changes in body composition occur. An adequate level of leptin appears to be permissive for sexual function, acting on neurons that secrete sex hormones.

Between women with normal menstrual cycles and those with amenorrhoea, leptin not only differs in its concentration, but also in its diurnal rhythm. These observations suggest that leptin probably signals energy availability rather than simply the state of the body's fat stores. This energy signalling is critical for reproductive function, as it ensures that the body has sufficient energy to support a potential pregnancy. The decrease in leptin in female athletes with AHF reflects an adaptation to a state of low energy availability, leading to suppression of reproductive function as an energy conservation measure [(7].

• Diagnosis

Making the diagnosis of FHA can be challenging, particularly at younger ages as this is often the time of HPO axis development. Primary amenorrhoea should always be ruled out, as 98% of girls will reach menarche by the age of 15. Furthermore, 90% of menstrual cycles will be between 21 and 45 days, even in the first few years after menarche, so it is important to investigate secondary amenorrhoea in adolescence. As FHA is a non-organic cause of amenorrhoea, it is considered a diagnosis of exclusion [1].

To reach a diagnosis, an exhaustive study must be carried out to rule out anatomical and organic causes of amenorrhoea. A correct anamnesis, physical examination, blood tests and radiological studies are essential [1].

•Treatment

Specifically, in amenorrheic athletes, a multidisciplinary approach is recommended including: nutritional therapy, psychological therapy and modification of training planning. Nutritional therapy focuses on ensuring adequate caloric intake to restore normal energy and hormonal function. Psychological therapy can help manage stress and underlying eating disorders. Training modification focuses on balancing exercise with recovery to avoid overtraining.

•Justification

Bearing in mind that, in the case of women, elite sport is still a very short journey, it is necessary to review the information on certain problems that compromise female athletes and that lead to menstrual problems, even reaching AHF. The aim of this review is to gather the most relevant information on the risk factors that can lead to this pathology in order to pay special attention to preventing it .

2. OBJECTIVES

The following are the objectives designed to be achieved in order carry out this work:

General objective:

• To learn about preventive nutritional measures and treatment of hypothalamic amenorrhoea in sportsmen and women athletes.

Specific objectives:

Based on the general objective formulated above, five specific objectives have been developed, from which it is intended to achieve a greater degree of detail on the subject addressed.

• To identify the characteristic signs and symptoms of this pathology for early detection.
• To know whether clear diagnostic criteria have been established that can help differentiate this pathology from others that also include cessation of menstruation such as PCOS.
• To determine which social factors influence the development of hypothalamic amenorrhoea in young female athletes.
• To investigate, through the available literature, which nutritional factors should be applied in the prevention of hypothalamic amenorrhoea in female athletes.
• To find out whether it might be beneficial to add some kind of supplement to the diet of sportswomen to prevent hypothalamic amenorrhoea.

At On the basis of a all of above, we question some questions research questions on the basis of which we will focus the bibliographical analysis.

Researchable questions:

SITUATION:

Patient: Women athletes.

Intervention/ comparison: Nutritional guidelines.

Outcomes: Cessation of amenorrhoea.

ISSUES TO BE ADDRESSED BY THE LITERATURE SEARCH

Are the triggers described so far for functional hypothalamic amenorrhoea correct?

What are the correct nutritional guidelines for the treatment Hypothalamic Amenorrhoea in female athletes?

Is energy intake in adolescence related to female athlete triad in adult female endurance athletes?

What nutritional deficits do female athletes with hypothalamic amenorrhoea have?

Where is the research to prevent or treat hypothalamic amenorrhoea in female athletes heading?

3. METHODOLOGY

This systematic review has been carried out following the PRISMA (Preferred Reporting Items for Systematic Reviews and Meta- Analysis) Statement (http://www.prisma-statement.org/), which promotes transparency in the presentation of systematic reviews and meta-analyses, ensuring that authors provide a full description of the methods and results of their research.

3.1. Bibliographic Search

The search strategy consisted of consulting, during the months of April and May 2021, the meta-search engine available in the Health Library of the Complejo Asitencial Universitario de León for professionals. The following databases were used: PubMed, Medline, Cinhal, Cochrane, Scopus and Web of Science. The descriptors "Women", "Amenorrhea", "Exercise", "Athletes" and "Nutrition" were used. The selection filters used were: Randomised clinical trials, Narrative/systematic review and Meta-analysis. In addition, we filtered those studies carried out from 2016 onwards with Full Text available in the library of the University Health Care Complex of León. Likewise, the works written in English and Spanish were selected.

3.2. Selection of studies

After carrying out the search, a total of 118 articles were found in the databases used. In order to close the number of articles that make up the study, the following process was carried out. Those studies that were found to be repeated were excluded, only one of them was repeated, so the search was reduced to 117 studies. Subsequently, we proceeded to read the summaries of the 117 studies, excluding those conducted in animals (2), those conducted in men and which were not relevant to the objective of this study or were not closely related to the specific subject of the review, for example, those conducted in strength athletes or those focused on obesity. Thus, 80 of the 117 studies obtained as a result of the search were excluded, leaving 37 of them. Of these 37 studies, a further 12 were excluded due to an excess of information on the psychological aspects of FHA.Finally, 25 studies were selected for critical reading to obtain the salient information from each of them. This reading was carried out by the same person, in order to avoid any possible bias in the choice of articles. On the other hand, the Reading was carried out in an exhaustive manner, completing a chek-list, which was drawn up for this purpose, ensuring that all the articles selected complied with the same methodological aspects.

3.3. Critical reading

The critical reading was carried out according to the Spanish Critical Appraisal Skills Programme CASPE (Programa de Habilidades en lectura Crítica Español). This is an educational programme designed to improve the skills of health professionals and others interested in critically appraising scientific research and evidence available in the medical and scientific literature. This programme aims to train participants to read, interpret and evaluate scientific studies, enabling them to make informed, evidence-based decisions.

Objectives of CASPe:

Fostering critical skills: helping participants to develop a critical and analytical mindset towards scientific information.

Improving clinical decision-making: facilitating the application of the best scientific evidence in daily clinical practice.

Promoting evidence-based practice: integrating the best available evidence with clinical experience and patient values.

3.4. Flowchart:

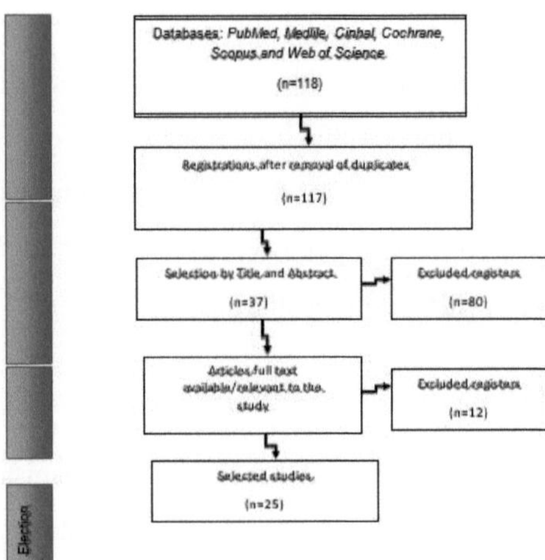

4. RESULTS

In this section, the results of the recent literature review on the impact of various supplements and nutritional strategies on athletic performance and general health will be discussed and developed. The review covers key studies exploring the efficacy of creatine supplementation, the benefits of probiotics, as well as the importance of essential nutrients such as omega-3, calcium and vitamin D in female athletes. Each of these elements is discussed in terms of their specific effects on athletic ability, recovery, and overall health, providing a comprehensive view of how these factors contribute to optimising performance and well-being. In addition, it will discuss how different dosing and supplementation strategies may influence outcomes and practical recommendations derived from the literature reviewed. This review aims to provide an in-depth understanding of best practices and evidence-based approaches to improve performance and health in the context of sport.

4.1. Triggering factors

Sophie Gibson et al. (2020) [(1)] conducted a review study on the assessment and management of Functional Hypothalamic Amenorrhoea (FHA). In their paper they describe the most important factors related to this pathology with special mention to those triggers of FHA such as Eating Disorders (ED), as FHA is often found to be the underlying aetiology of patients with suspected ED due to their amenorrhoea condition but who maintain a normal weight and therefore do not meet clear criteria for ED. On the other hand, disordered eating is quite common in adolescent-aged women, which makes diagnosis even more difficult. This study also indicates that women with FHA show greater cognitive restraint, drive for thinness and purging behaviours than eumenorrhoeic women. The onset of amenorrhoea is also related to stressful situations indicating that 50% of these women suffer from family conflicts. It is also mentioned that patients with FHA cope worse with stress compared to those with PCOS or eumenorrhoeic women. Another trigger, the most prominent in this review, is excessive exercise; Gibson et al. note that rates of ALF are three times higher in female athletes, with long-distance runners being particularly affected. In addition, they suggest that there may be a genetic basis for the development of ALF, six heterozygous genetic mutations can be identified (FGFR fibroblast growth factor receptor 1 gene, PROKR2 prokineticin receptor 2 gene, PROKR2 prokineticin receptor 1 gene, FGFR fibroblast growth factor receptor 1 gene, PROKR2 prokineticin receptor 2 gene, FGFR prokineticin receptor 2 gene), GnRH receptor gene GNRHR and Kallamnn Syndrome 1 sequence gene KAL 1) in patients with FHA that are common to patients with Congenital Hypogonadotropic Hypogonadism, suggesting a possible heightened vulnerability to stressors on the HPO axis [(1)].

Table 1: Hormone pattern in AHF [(1)]

Hormone	Level
Pituitary	
FSH	Low
LH	Low
TSH	Low-Normal
PRL	Normal
Ovarian	
Estradiol	Low
Testosterone	Low-Normal
AMH	Normal

FSH: follicle stimulating hormone, LH: luteinizing hormone, TSH: thyroid-stimulating hormone, PRL: prolactin, AMH: anti-Müllerian hormone. Ref. 11,12,13,14,41,42.

In addition to those already mentioned in this study, weight loss is important as a triggering factor, which should also be a fundamental piece of information in the diagnosis, during the anamnesis and physical examination of the patient. If weight loss is identified as a contributing factor, it is important to consider the weight at which the patient started amenorrhoea and the rate of weight loss. It is important to investigate how this weight loss occurred, as this will help to differentiate from ACT [(1)].

•Sport y health: Disorders from Eating behaviour eating disorders (ED):

Eating disorders (EDs) are serious psychological conditions that affect a person's relationship with food and body image. The most common EDs include anorexia nervosa, bulimia nervosa and binge eating disorder. These disorders can have devastating physical and mental health consequences, including malnutrition, damage to vital organs, depression and anxiety. In the sports context, the prevalence of EDD is particularly high due to the pressure to maintain certain physical standards, especially in sports that emphasise leanness or specific weight, such as gymnastics, athletics, dance and combat sports. Athletes may develop disordered eating behaviours in an effort to improve their performance or achieve the aesthetic ideal promoted in their discipline. The pressure to reach "ideal weight" or maintain low body fat can lead to unhealthy behaviours, such as extreme calorie restriction, excessive use of dietary supplements, and compulsive exercise. These practices not only compromise athletic performance, but also put the athlete's overall health at risk. Furthermore, EDCs in sport are often underdiagnosed due to the lack of adequate screening tools and the tendency to normalise dangerous practices in certain sport environments. For this reason, it is crucial to develop prevention and early detection strategies, as well as to provide adequate psychological and nutritional support to athletes to promote a healthy relationship with food and the body.The review study by Xantophoulos et al. (2020) [(2)], refers to the mental problems that can most affect the young sports population, including depression, anxiety, ADHD (Attention Deficit Hyperactivity Disorder), psychoactive substance use and EDD [((1,2)).] It is worth noting in this review that EDD affects the athlete population to a greater extent than the non-athlete population and that it affects women to a much greater extent, with men comprising between 10% and 25% of people with EDD [(2)].It is noteworthy in the study [(2)], that characteristics associated with the mindset of an elite athlete (e.g., focus on performance, perfection and control) in combination with the context of the sporting environment are associated with eating pathology, body dissatisfaction and compulsive exercise. Furthermore, they add that athletes may have a "normal" weight and may not meet the exact diagnostic criteria for EDC because training contributes to increased muscle mass. The term "anorexia athletica" has coined to describe this phenomenon. Excessive exercise" is difficult to define in young elite athletes, however, there is clearly a threshold where the risks and negative outcomes outweigh the performance benefits (2).

Tranoulis et al. (2020) (3), conducted a prospective case-control study conducted from January 2016 to April 2018 with 41 women with ADHF and 86 healthy controls. They assessed disordered eating behaviours and other predisposing factors for ADHF using self-reported questionnaires. Their findings were that disordered eating behaviours were significantly more frequent in women with FHA (1,2,3). In addition, women with FHA were characterised by significantly higher scores on items of the subscale of specific dieting and preoccupation with food compared to healthy controls. Significant differences were also observed between the mean scores of the two groups on all other questionnaires. Their conclusion was that disordered eating behaviours may occur in FHA populations more frequently compared to the general population (1,2,3). Furthermore, they add that anxiety and preoccupation with being overweight may independently underlie and contribute to the development and maintenance of both these behaviours and FHA (3).

Mancine et al. (2020) (4), in their review of the prevalence of ED in the athlete population, investigated which factors influence this association and which sports are at highest risk. They add that research on aesthetic or weight-dependent sports found that athletes participating in these sports had significantly higher rates of disordered eating than those participating in non-aesthetic sports. In one of the studies they reviewed, the different sports did not have a statistically significant difference in eating disorder rates. However, when divided into "lean" and "non-lean" categories, the difference between the two categories is highly significant. They point out that, while there is clear evidence that emphasis on leanness plays an important role, when further subdivided into sports, the evidence is less concise. This means that, although useful, the grouping investigated so far does not provide a complete picture to address the risk of EDD [(4)]. In the clinical trial by Petisco et al. (2020) [(5)], once again reference is made to the risk of eating disorders in the athlete population [(1,2,3,4,5)] and the importance of identifying risk factors to better target prevention and intervention strategies [((5)).] These authors, in addition to referring to body image, add other factors such as pressure from coaches, parents and peers to lose weight, as well as a specific personality of athletes [((1,5)).] As already added by Mancine et al. [(4)], the risk varies according to gender, sport discipline and competitive level and is more prevalent in the female population and in the young population [(2,4)] (90% occur in people under the age of 18).25 years of age). They point to a possible higher prevalence in athletes than in the general population [(4,5)], but there is insufficient evidence as there are studies that point to the contrary. They add typical personality characteristics of the elite athlete, such as perfectionism, which is desirable for sporting success, but adds to the risk of ED [(2,5)]; it is also linked to a certain level of anxiety; low self-esteem also seems to be important for body image dissatisfaction, although it is difficult to know whether this is a cause or an effect of it. The study by Petisco et al., [((5))] [consisted] of a sample of 120 professional athletes and non-athletes aged 15-25 years grouped into gymnasts, footballers and non-athletes. The assessment protocol consisted of five questionnaires, which were completed voluntarily, anonymously, individually and confidentially by the participants to analyse self-esteem, perfectionism, anxiety and the risk of developing eating disorders. In this study, they found that 2.5% of gymnasts, 12.5% of football players and 20% of non-athletes demonstrated disordered eating attitudes [(5)]. Therefore, it has shown a higher prevalence of disordered attitudes in the non-athlete population compared to the sports modalities studied [5]. They add that this result may be due to false answers from athletes.In the review study carried out by Kalindjian et al., (2021) [(6)], they carry out a review of secondary prevention in the sports population through early detection by the environment in which coaches find themselves. They point out that the majority of sports professionals feel involved in this type of detection, providing the following conclusions: almost all athletic trainers thought that their role was to identify EDs, while female trainers were more concerned about this problem. More than half of the coaches were interested in further training to facilitate early detection and all agreed to receive any recommendations on the subject. As far as FHA is concerned, this review refers to a study that notes that more than one third of sports coaches thought that amenorrhoea in an athlete was always normal. They also mention that only 10% of fitness coaches in Canada and Norway thought they could talk to a young woman about this issue. Furthermore, about two thirds of the elite coaches said they would contact the athlete to report that they had observed symptoms of ACT, but only 1/9 would refer them to a specialist [6].

4.2. Diagnosis of FHA

• Anamnesis

Anamnesis is a fundamental tool in the diagnosis of AHF in female athletes, as it provides a comprehensive view of the factors that may be contributing to the disruption of the menstrual cycle. AHF is a condition where stress, weight loss and intense exercise affect hormonal regulation, leading to the absence of menstruation. In female athletes, this condition is particularly prevalent due to the physical and psychological demands of their training. A detailed anamnesis allows the physician to assess multiple aspects of the patient's life, including dietary habits, level and type of physical activity, and emotional and psychological factors. Specific questions about diet may reveal nutritional deficits or underlying eating disorders, while inquiring about the workout regimen may highlight levels of exercise that negatively affect menstrual health. In addition, anamnesis can identify signs of stress and other psychosocial factors that contribute to AHF. This comprehensive assessment is essential to differentiate AHF from other causes of amenorrhoea, such as endocrine or anatomical problems, and to design a personalised treatment plan that addresses both the physical and emotional health of the patient. Gibson et al.[1] give special importance to the diagnostic section of FHA due to its complexity, they recommend starting with a clinical history where aspects such as family history and pathological history, use of medications; type of exercise, duration and intensity; if there is disordered eating, a dietary record may be useful; sexual history and use of contraceptives, triggers (stress, weight loss and excessive exercise) should be asked about. It is advisable to ask about signs of hyperandrogenism such as acne or hirsutism that could indicate PCOS or late onset Congenital Adrenal Hyperplasia. Vasomotor symptoms such as hot flushes may indicate primary ovarian insufficiency and symptoms of cyclic or chronic abdominal pain may point to a Müllerian abnormality [1].

• Blood test

The inclusion of a blood test in the diagnosis of Functional Hypothalamic Amenorrhoea (FHA) in female athletes is crucial for several reasons. reasons. Firstly, it allows assessment of the patient's hormonal status, including FSH and LH levels, oestrogen and prolactin, which is essential to confirm the diagnosis of AHF and to rule out other causes of amenorrhoea, such as thyroid disorders or hyperprolactinaemia.

In addition, blood work can identify nutritional deficiencies common in female athletes with AHF, such as low levels of iron, vitamin D, and calcium, which may contribute to menstrual dysfunction and other health problems. Assessing markers of stress and adrenal function, such as cortisol, also provides valuable information on the impact of intense training and stress on the hypothalamic-pituitary-ovarian axis.Detection of metabolic imbalances, such as alterations in glucose and insulin levels, may indicate the presence of insulin resistance or metabolic syndrome, conditions that can also affect menstrual function. Finally, a complete blood work-up helps establish a baseline to monitor response to treatment and adjust nutritional and training interventions as needed. It has been described as some of the parameters that should be included as a minimum are the measurement of Beta Subunit of GnRH concentration. In addition, they add the need to include FSH, LH, oestradiol, prolactin and TSH concentration, total and free testosterone, androstenedione and 17-hydroxyprogesterone in the early morning. They also suggest cortisol measurement [(1)].

• Radiological tests

According to Gibson et al. [(1)], ultrasound of the pelvis will be necessary to identify the presence of the uterus and ovaries, as well as to rule out the existence of an adnexal mass, which could be indicative of other gynaecological pathologies. This evaluation is essential to confirm the normal anatomy of the reproductive tract and to exclude other structural causes of amenorrhoea. In addition, due to the significant risk of developing osteopenia and osteoporosis associated with prolonged hypoestrogenism, bone mineral density assessment by dual-energy X-ray absorptiometry (DEXA/DXA) is highly recommended in patients presenting with prolonged amenorrhoea. DEXA/DXA is an accurate and reliable tool to measure bone density and detect any decrease that may predispose to fractures. It may also be useful to complement this study with a lateral spine X-ray to evaluate possible asymptomatic vertebral fractures, which are common in women with low oestrogen levels. long-term. Early detection of these fractures allows for timely intervention and may prevent future complications. Together, these diagnostic tests not only help to identify and confirm the diagnosis of functional hypothalamic amenorrhoea, but also provide a comprehensive assessment of the systemic impact of this condition, thus guiding more effective and personalised clinical management to protect patients' bone and overall health [((10))].

4.3. Treatment: Lifestyle modification

This review [1] points to lifestyle modification as the primary treatment for AHF. Women with FHA, especially those whose condition is associated with significant weight loss, should be managed comprehensively by a healthcare team, with a special focus on nutrition. It is essential that these patients receive ongoing nutritional care for at least six months to address dietary deficiencies and promote healthy weight gain. The data presented in this review are revealing: 54% of treated patients were able to resume their menstrual cycle within an average period of 19±5 months. This result underlines the importance of prolonged and consistent follow-up.One of the key findings is the increase in body mass index (BMI) in these women prior to resumption of menstruation. Although the increase was small, it was statistically significant, indicating that even a modest increase in BMI can have a positive impact on the restoration of menstrual function. The general recommendation for women with FHA is a weight gain of approximately 1-2 kg, or 5% of initial body weight. This not only helps to resume menstruation, but has also been shown to improve bone mineral density (BMD), a crucial factor for long-term bone health.In addition to nutritional recommendations, the importance of calcium and vitamin D supplementation to support bone health in women with FHA is emphasised. Between 1200-1500 mg of calcium per day, along with 400-1000 IU of vitamin D, is recommended. This supplementation is vital to prevent osteopenia and osteoporosis, common conditions in women with low oestrogen levels due to FHA. Adequate supplementation not only helps maintain bone health, but can also speed recovery of menstrual function. The review also highlights the importance of psychological therapy as an integral part of the treatment for the FHA. The stress is a factor.significant which may contribute to hypothalamic dysfunction and subsequent amenorrhoea. Therefore, psychological therapy aimed at improving stress coping skills is essential. Psychoeducation, a form of therapy that educates patients about the relationship between stress and their condition, has shown promising results in recent studies. The implementation of this therapy has no known harmful effects on patients and can provide valuable tools for managing stress effectively.In conclusion, management of AHF should be multifaceted, addressing both nutritional and psychological aspects. Lifestyle modification, including weight gain and appropriate supplementation, along with psychological therapy, can lead to successful resumption of menstrual function and improved bone health. Comprehensive and personalised care based on the individual needs of each patient is fundamental to the effective treatment of FHA [(1)].

They add that research on pharmacological treatment in FHA aims to promote improved bone health and prevent the development of osteoporosis. Transdermal estrogen therapy appears to be promising according to this study, as lack of estrogen during the premenopausal years has been associated with decreased BMD. Further research is needed on new lines of treatment with recombinant human leptin and kisspeptin [((1).] In the review study by Hirsberg et al. (2020) [(7)] on female hyperandrogenism and elite sport, they emphasise the higher prevalence of amenorrhoea in elite athletes [(1,7)], particularly in those where a slim body is considered an advantage for physical performance, such as in aesthetic and endurance sports [((1,2,3,4,7)).] They suggest that the most important underlying cause for the development of this problem is an energy deficit relative to caloric expenditure sometimes due to the desire to be thin. A relatively low amount of body fat relative to muscle mass is important for performance in many disciplines, including athletics [(7)]. At the same time, these authors point out that strict control of food intake can lead to ED, which is more prevalent in the athletic population than in the general population [((1-7)).]

Furthermore, they point out the paradox that, given that physical activity promotes bone formation, it is curious that these elite athletes had reduced BMD. It is now known that this phenomenon arises from nutritional deficiency and its endocrine consequences including low levels of oestradiol, testosterone and IGF-I, as well as elevated cortisol [(1,7)]. They add that AHF is a reversible condition that can be reversed by restoring the balance between intake and energy expenditure, as noted by Gibson et al [((1))]. They add that if nutritional counselling and adjustment of training for at least one year does not lead to resumption of menstruation, estrogen drug therapy may be considered [(7)].

4.4. Polycystic Ovary Syndrome (PCOS)

Although low energy availability is the most common cause of amenorrhoea among female athletes [(7)], not all athletes with menstrual disorders are hypometabolic. In fact, Hirsberg et al. identify PCOS as an alternative explanation. PCOS is probably the most prevalent endocrine disorder in women of childbearing age, affecting 10% of the female population. It is characterised by elevated ovarian androgen production, impaired ovulation and ultrasound findings of polycystic ovaries. Although its aetiology is still unknown, there are indications of a genetic predisposition. The characteristic endocrine features of PCOS are insulin resistance and hyperandrogenism which explain the associated symptoms. The clinical consequences are the characteristic polycystic ovarian morphology and anovulation leading to menstrual disorders and reduced fertility, as well as hirsutism and acne. Furthermore, these authors add that women with PCOS are more insulin resistant, independent of obesity, leading to a secondary hypersecretion of insulin, which directly stimulates androgen production by ovarian theca cells. Also, insulin inhibits hepatic synthesis of sex hormone binding globulin (SHBG), thereby elevating free and bioavailable testosterone levels. Insulin resistance can lead to abdominal obesity [(7)]. Treatment of this condition is managed by treating the symptoms, including menstrual disorders, infertility, hirsutism and overweight/obesity. The mainstay is a healthy lifestyle [1,7], including regular physical activity. In addition, combined oral contraceptives androgenic effects and counteract hirsutism and acne. Physical activity generally improves fertility in women with PCOS(7). In this review [7], we can also read that PCOS is a common disorder among elite female athletes and is, in fact, the most frequent cause of menstrual disorders among Olympic athletes. To differentiate from FHA, we see that in PCOS there is an elevated diurnal secretion of LH and testosterone. In contrast, in athletes with AIH due to energy deficiency, LH pulsatility is nullified and testosterone levels are low [(1,7)]. Therefore, the hormone profile associated with the SOP differs completely from FHA. It should be noted that the physique of athletes with PCOS is more anabolic, with a greater amount of muscle mass and greater bone mineral density than other athletes. In addition, they point out that PCOS is related to a better VO2max and that it can favour performance, something that does not happen in FHA. Thus, they conclude that mild forms of hyperandrogenism, such as PCOS, may improve physical performance and therefore play a role in women's decision to engage in sport, which may explain the higher incidence of PCOS in female athletes than in sedentary women. There is no evidence that sporting activities promote hyperandrogenism [7].

Figure 2: Differential diagnosis of AHF.

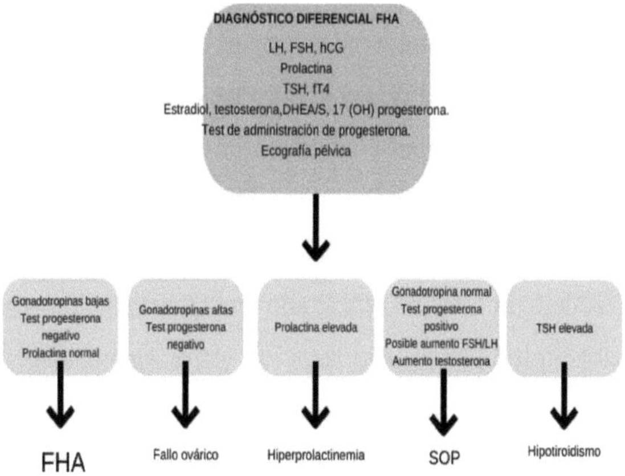

4.5. Hormonal responses to excessive exercise

Given that intense exercise is a trigger for AHF [(1)], Melin et al. (2019) [(8)] conducted a cohort study of athletes eumenorrheic (control) and FHA on the impact of menstrual function in relation to intense physical activity. Athletes aged 18-38 years were selected from the Danish team and Swedish endurance sports federations (middle and long distance, orienteering and triathlon), and through local sports clubs in the Oresund region (Denmark) and Sweden. Two incremental exercise tests (T^1 and T^2) were performed on a cycloergometer with four hours of recovery in between, at 11.00 and 15.00 hours, two hours after breakfast. and lunch containing no more than 650 kcal, respectively. The tests were started by pedalling for 6 min at 50 watts, followed by increasing the workload from 12 to 14 watts per minute until exhaustion, with a cadence of 60 rpm. The results of this study were that athletes with FHA had lower total body mass and fat mass compared to controls, but no differences in aerobic capacity were found. In addition, athletes with FHA had a lower percentage of fat-free mass than controls. In relation to endocrine responses, Melin et al. [(8)], concluded that there were no differences in hormone response after the first exercise session; however, after the second test, IGFBP-3 increased more in FHA with a similar trend for IGF-1 and DBNF which were not considered significant. Lombardi et al., (2020) [9] conducted a review study focusing on parathyroid hormone (PTH) regulation and physical activity-dependent calcium-phosphorus metabolism. They concluded that changes in circulating PTH levels during and after exercise are dependent on duration and/or intensity; these researchers hypothesise that the PTH response is activated when a threshold in intensity and duration is exceeded. In general, they add that marked increases in PTH are observed only for high intensity and duration (15% above ventilatory threshold for more than 50 minutes) or for low intensity and very long duration (50% VO_2 max more than 5 hours). In case of short series of very short duration (30 seconds) at maximum intensity there is no effect on PTH secretion. The increase occurs in the late phase of long-duration exercise and in the recovery phase. Furthermore, the exercise-induced increase in PTH appears to be partially driven by an exercise-induced increase in calcium levels [9]. A low level of physical activity, together with limited calcium intake, is associated with an increased risk of PTH disturbance. Optimal physical activity status together with dietary supplementation (calcium and/or vitamin D) may be beneficial to health. However, it is posible that such supplementation must be combined with exercise to be effective [9].

4.6. Hormonal contraception and sports performance

Elliot-Sale et al. [10], in their meta-analysis of whether the use of hormonal contraception improves or worsens performance, concluded that performance was slightly higher in women who did not use hormonal contraception and who had regular menstrual cycles. Taken together, their findings indicate that OCPs may have a relatively negative impact on performance; but, from a practical point of view, the decision on the appropriateness of OCP use should be tailored to individual requirements. As a result of OCP use, endogenous oestradiol and progesterone concentrations are lower compared to the average luteal phase of the menstrual cycle without OCP. This chronic down-regulation may be responsible for the slightly impaired exercise performance demonstrated in OCP users compared to those who menstruate naturally. In fact, the endogenous hormone profile of an OCP user is comparable to the profile observed during the early follicular phase of the physiological menstrual cycle, i.e. low levels of endogenous oestradiol and progesterone. Taken together, these results indicate that exercise performance may be mediated by the concentration of endogenous ovarian hormones in some individuals [(10)].

4.7. Physical activity and infertility

Research by Dhair et al. (2020) [(11)] explored the association between type, intensity and frequency of physical activity with primary infertility in an analytical observational case-control study involving 320 women in Gaza. This study revealed significant findings on how different exercise patterns affect the female reproductive hormonal axis. The results indicate that the relationship between physical activity and women's reproductive health can be both beneficial and detrimental, depending on a number of factors, such as the type of activity, its frequency and intensity. The study concluded that an optimal level regular exercise is crucial for maintaining substantial overall health benefits. However, women who undergo intense and prolonged exercise are at increased risk of experiencing reproductive health-related problems. These women are more likely to develop amenorrhoea, either primary or secondary, which can negatively affect their fertility. Amenorrhoea is a condition in which the menstrual cycle is disrupted, which can complicate conception and reproductive ability.In addition, the study found that women who participate in intense physical activity from an early age are more likely to experience a delay in menarche, which is the first onset of menstruation. This delayed menarche may have long-term implications for women's reproductive health and hormonal development. The analysis also identified several additional variables associated with primary infertility. There was a significant positive association between primary infertility and factors such as age at marriage over 28 years, menarche occurring before age 14, as well as poverty and refugee status. These social and economic factors may interrelate with the effects of physical activity and contribute to infertility.Dhair et al. (2020) also noted that sedentary lifestyle, or lack of physical activity, is another important risk factor for infertility. In contrast, women who are normal weight, even if they engage in intense physical activity, have a lower risk of menstrual disturbances compared to those who are overweight or obese. This suggests that body weight status and exercise intensity should be considered together to assess the risk of infertility and other reproductive problems(11).

4.8. Socio-cultural considerations

Heather et al. (2021) (12) conducted a cross-sectional survey of 219 elite female athletes in New Zealand, which aimed to quantify the health status of elite female athletes and to understand the socio-cultural factors that influence health status. A total of 357 elite female athletes from New Zealand were recruited to complete a survey. 219 of these completed the survey. 22% met the criteria for late menarche, only 2 of the respondents required intervention (medication, weight gain, reduced training load) to initiate menstruation. 63% were not using hormonal contraceptives, of which 13% had amenorrhoea. A previous diagnosis of oligo- or amenorrhoea was positively associated with a history of stress fractures and eating disorders. Thirty-seven percent were users of hormonal contraception. The combined hormonal contraceptive pill was most frequently used for contraception, but also for menstrual control, regularity, symptom reduction, and acne. Fifty-six percent reported side effects on mood and weight gain (12). The majority of female athletes reported menstrual cycle symptoms (Table 4).

Table 2: Characteristics of the menstrual cycle [12]

Menstrual cycle characteristic	n	Respondents	Percent
Regularity (when not using hormonal contraception)			
Regular	111	206	54
Not regular	32	206	16
Don't know/Other	63	206	31
Menstrual cycle-related symptoms			
Pelvic pain	115	202	57
Increased fatigue	99	202	49
Low back pain	94	202	47
Disrupted sleep	58	202	29
Headaches	39	202	19
Pain in thighs	20	202	10
Nausea or vomiting	17	202	8
Other	46	202	23
Nil	41	202	20
Requiring pain relief during menstruation			
Never	65	203	32
Rarely	72	203	35
Most of time	54	203	27
Always	12	203	6
Menstrual period characteristics			
Considered heavy	60	203	30
Not considered heavy	146	203	72
Need to frequently change pads or tampons	50	201	25
Passing large blood clots	42	201	21
Flooding through protection	34	201	17
Required to use double sanitary protection	17	201	8
Struggle to complete training without changing sanitary protection	18	201	8

One-third of female athletes reported that their menstrual cycle was affected by training volume. Thirty-six per cent believed that their menstrual cycle negatively impacted their performance while 28% believed that performance was not affected by their menstrual cycle. Four per cent believed that their menstrual cycle had a positive impact on performance. 86% reported that they were not absent from their training because of menstruation [12]. Also in the survey by Heather et al. (2021) [12] questions about social pressure on female athletes were included. The results were that 73 % of the athletes felt that their sport was putting pressure on them to change their appearance which they believed was detrimental to their health. Social media was the most recognised source of pressure. 33 of the athletes reported engaging in disordered eating practices to obtain the "ideal" body and 22 reported being told by their coach to lose weight for performance-related reasons. 1 in 3 reported that they had never received any health-related information. Eighty percent reported that there was no barrier to communication, however, barriers observed included when the coach, doctor and other support professionals were male, as there was a perceived lack of knowledge and stigmatisation of the issue [12].

4.9. Female Athlete Triad/ Relative Energy Deficiency in Sport (RED-S)

Since the early 1990s, the Female Athlete Triad has been used to describe female athletes who also have eating disorders, amenorrhoea and low bone mineral density [1,13, (14)]. In 2017, The American College of Obstetricians and Gynecologists revised this terminology to be more inclusive. The current criteria are: Low energy availability with or without eating disorder, menstrual dysfunction and low bone mineral density [1,14]. This term differs from FHA because it is not necessary for the athlete to be amenorrheic to meet the triad criteria. Not all patients with FHA are athletes or meet the Triad criteria. All female athletes are at risk for this problem [14], regardless of body build or sport. All active women should be assessed for the components of the triad and additional assessments should be conducted if one or more components are identified. Using the menstrual cycle as a vital sign is a useful tool to identify women at risk and should be an integral part of the sports physical examination prior to training and competition planning [14].In the review study by Williams et al. (2019) [15], the conceptual representation of the Female Athlete Triad and Relative Energy Deficiency in Sport in Figures 6 and 7 [15] is noteworthy.

Figure 3: Illustration of the aspects of the triad of the female athlete [15]

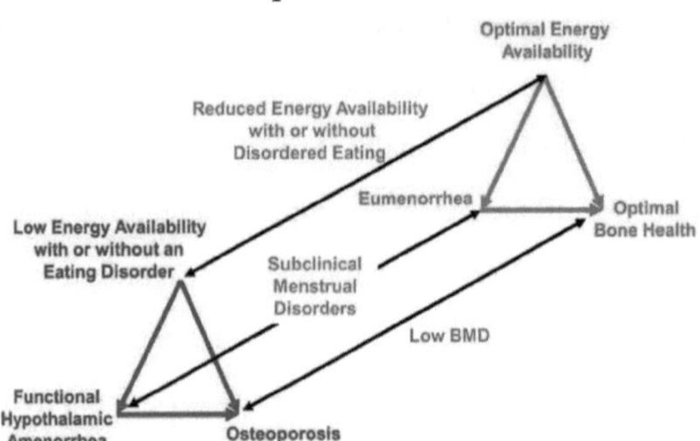

In the image you can see the three interrelated components of the female athlete Triad which are energy availability, menstrual status and bone health [1,13,14,15]. Energy availability directly affects menstrual status and, in turn, energy availability and menstrual status directly bone health. Optimal health is indicated by optimal energy availability, eumenorrhoea and optimal bone health, while at the other end of the picture, the most severe form of the female athlete's triad is characterised by low energy availability with or without an eating disorder, FHA and osteoporosis [(15)].

Figure 4: Health Consequences of Relative Energy in Sport (RED-S). [15]

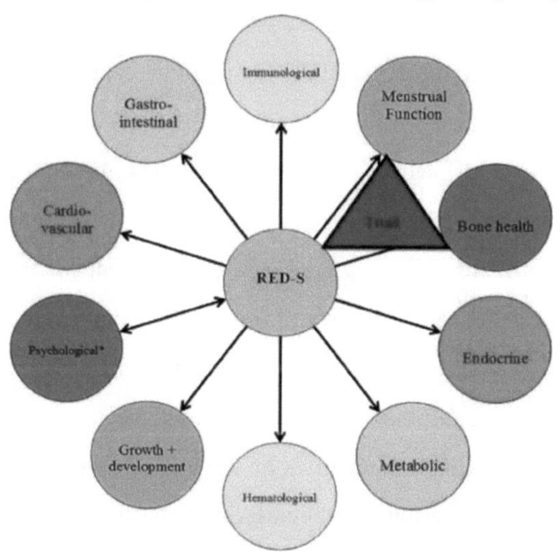

Figure 7 [15] represents an expanded view of the Female Athlete Triad to illustrate a wider range of outcomes and application to male athletes. These authors stress that RED-S should not be considered as a diagnosable condition or as an evidence-based syndrome, rather it should be considered as a concept, as was once the case with the Triad which will need extensive discussion, debate and experimentation [(15)].De Souza et al., (2017) [16], in their review to assess the current status of the female athlete Triad, highlight several aspects such as that female athletes suffering from the Triad often present one or more of the three components of the Triad, and the presence of one is sufficient to diagnose it [(14,15)]. It is important to recognise that each component of the Triad presents along a continuum from a healthy starting point to an unhealthy point of severity (see figure 6). In addition, progression through the three phases can occur at different rates. He adds that subsequent to the Triad an alternative was proposed called Relative Energy Deficiency in Sport (RED-S) which is described as a wheel (see figure 7) in which energy deficiency acts as the central hub. These authors point out that this model is incorrect as it suggests that energy deficiency exerts direct effects on many different systems not included in the fundamental Triad model [(15)]. For example, the RED-S model inaccurately describes a direct relationship between energy deficit and endothelial dysfunction when it is correct that energy deficiency suppresses the reproductive axis which has downstream effects on vascular function. These authors therefore warn against the strict adoption of the RES-S model as a replacement for the female athlete triad. In reference to reproductive health they add that disorders associated with the triad include severe menstrual disorders such as amenorrhoea and subclinical disorders defined as luteal phase defects and anovulation. In addition, they note that optimal menstrual function depends on the availability of fuel. They include mention of research exploring neuroendocrine links between nutritional status and reproductive function, adding that several studies identify leptin as a key signal for the hypothalamic reproductive axis. In relation leptin, in the clinical trial by Moskvicheva et al. [(18)], an assessment of nutritional status, anthropometry, eating disorders, fat tissue and leptin levels was performed in 48 patients with FHA. The nutritional status study revealed discrepancy between caloric intake and energy expenditure in 50% of patients, inadequate carbohydrate intake in 91.7%, high protein intake in 70.8% of patients. In addition, weight loss was observed in 29.2% of patients, body fat in 100% of patients with low BMI and in 58.8% with normal BMI. Decreased leptin levels were detected in 77.1% of patients and hypercholesterolaemia without an increase in the atherogenic index in 68.8% of patients [(18)].

4.10. Reduction of Bone Mineral Density (BMD)

Bone mineral density (BMD) is crucial for sportsmen and athletes as it directly influences bone health and fracture prevention. Adequate BMD ensures that bones are strong and able to withstand the recurring stresses and impacts associated with training and competition. Athletes participating in high-impact sports, such as athletics, basketball or football, are at an increased risk of fractures if their bone density is insufficient. In addition, adequate BMD is essential for the prevention of osteoporosis and other degenerative bone diseases. Athletes with low bone mineral density may face an increased risk of stress fractures, which are common in sports involving high repetitive loads. Regular BMD monitoring helps to identify deficiencies and take preventive or corrective measures, such as adjustments in nutrition, training, and calcium and vitamin D supplementation.

BMD also impacts athletic performance; strong, healthy bones allow for faster recovery and greater resistance to physical exertion. Therefore, maintaining optimal bone mineral density is not only crucial for an athlete's overall health, but also to ensure a prolonged and successful athletic career.

The purpose of the clinical trial by Southmayd et al. (2016) [(19)], was to describe BMD and estimated bone geometry in exercising women (n = 60) grouped according to energy status and oestrogen status, resulting in four distinct groups. This study describes bone characteristics in young, physically active women as a function of energy and oestrogen status, demonstrating that these factors exert combined and independent effects on BMD, bone geometry and estimated bone strength. The results were that the combination of an energy deficiency and an oestrogen deficiency is more detrimental to bone than either deficiency alone and, given that energy deficiency often precedes menstrual disturbances in exercising women, treating hypoestrogenism without treating the malnutrition aspect of energy deficiency is likely to be insufficient to preserve or restore bone health. These data provide further evidence that adequate energy and healthy menstrual function should be health priorities in young exercising women (19).

In the review study by Papageorgiou et al. (2018) (20) they add that energy deficiency, in the short term, can increase markers of bone resorption and decrease markers of bone formation in active women. In the long term, they add that energy deficiency will lead to lower bone mass, impaired metabolism, increased risk of injury and stress fractures (20).

Ogwumike et al. (2018) (21) conducted a study to investigate the association between menstrual cycle status and musculoskeletal problems through a cross-sectional survey of female athletes in Nigeria. Participants were purposively sampled. From this investigation they concluded a prevalence of 24.9%. of menstrual irregularities in the participants, of whom 15.4% and 9.5% suffered from oligomenorrhoea and amenorrhoea respectively. The overall 12-month prevalence of menstrual disorders was 56.6%. The prevalence of menstrual disorders among participants reporting menstrual irregularity was 81.1% and 69.6%, respectively, for oligomenorrhoea and amenorrhoea. It was observed that amenorrhoeic athletes had a higher number of absences from sports participation for more than 30 days due to major menstrual disorders. There was a significant association between menstrual cycle status and musculoskeletal problems among female athletes in Nigeria (21).

Wasserfurth et al. (2017) (22) note that female runners with FHA have lower oestrogen levels (19,22); as a consequence, rapid bone loss is associated with menstrual disorders. The risk of bone fracture in amenorrhoeic elite female runners is nine times higher than that of their healthy counterparts. In women, oestradiol levels are extremely sensitive to LEA. Oestradiol preserves BMD by increasing osteoclasts and decreasing osteoblast apoptosis. The influence of LEA on BMD is evident in the analysis bone turnover markers. They mention that changes were found in three bone turnover markers in response to short-term ASF in exercising women, a reduction in the bone formation markers plasma osteocalcin and carboxy-terminal propeptide of procollagen type I in blood, and an increase in the bone resorption marker N-terminal telopeptide in urine. Extreme LEA (10 kcal/kg FFM/day) increased markers of bone resorption, while markers of bone formation decreased at lower levels of energy restriction between 20-30 kcal (22).

The review study by Southmayd et al (2017) (23) shows that the bone loss associated with the triad cannot always be fully recovered after a period of chronic LEA and hypoestrogenism· They indicate that amenorrhoeic athletes have 2% to 17% lower BMD in the lumbar spine than eumenorrhoeic athletes. Bone health biases in women affected by the triad also include unfavourable adaptations in bone geometry; women with menstrual irregularity are three times more likely to have a low femoral neck cross-sectional area. They add that geometry, microarchitecture and estimated strength are also compromised. In addition, bone benefits were seen in eumenorrhoeic but not amenorrhoeic athletes. This study suggests that menstrual regularity implies healthy oestrogen environment and adequate energy (19, 22, 23) to protect bone health, which implies a lower risk of fractures. In female athletes, stress fractures are a major concern, with an incidence of 9.2% in all female athletes, but may be higher than 20% in athletes in lean sports such as track and field. Importantly, a recent assessment of the cumulative effect of triad risk factors on the incidence of bone stress injuries revealed that having a low BMD and a BMI <21.0 kg/m^2 resulted in a 4.7-fold increase in the risk of bone stress injuries, which increased to a 6.8-fold increased risk if the athlete trained at least 12 hours per week (23).In this review (23), they mention that, in a one-year follow-up study of low BMD in amenorrhoeic female runners, female runners who resumed menstruation had gained 1.9 kg, coinciding with a significant increase of 0.071 g/cm^2 in BMD of the lumbar spine, compared to the additional decreases in BMD observed in female runners who remained amenorrhoeic. In particular, runners who had resumed menstruation still had a BMD 13% lower than that of runners who were eumenorrhoeic at baseline, highlighting that the potential for bone recovery may be limited, and that the time course of bone recovery is longer than that of energy and menstrual recovery [(23)].

4.11. Treatment options for poor bone health

Since there is a direct relationship between weight gain and increased BMD, nutritional interventions are the most logical treatment and first line of therapy for the triad because this strategy targets the aetiology of the syndrome: chronic energy deficiency.

According to Southmayd et al (2017) [(23)], the guidelines detail the need for a multidisciplinary approach, with an approach through improved energy intake and nutrition education by a dietitian. For more severe eating disorders, assessment and treatment requires a physician, a sports dietitian and a mental health professional. If after one year of treatment, reversal of energy deficiency is not achieved, if there is no reduction in BMD z-score or new fractures occur, pharmacological strategies should be considered in addition to nutritional treatment plans. Pharmacological strategies will be directed towards hypoestrogenism with combined oral contraceptive therapy. According to this study, 92% of sports medicine specialists and family physicians have prescribed OCP therapy to increase BMD in amenorrhoeic athletes. In conclusion, addressing both oestrogenic and energetic factors with appropriate treatment is of utmost importance [(23)].

4.12. Nutritional considerations for prevention

Wasserfurth et al. (2017) [22], in their review study, observed that, in healthy women, lower leptin levels are entirely dependent on energy availability, but are also a response to long-term physical training. They note that, when energy availability is less than 30 kcal/kg LBM/day, leptin is reduced at 24 hours, decreasing the Basal Metabolic Rate (BMR), inhibiting thyroid function, the reproductive and growth axis and the inflammatory response. They note that in studies of sedentary women of normal weight, 45 Kcal/kg BMR/day was presented as a threshold at which optimal energy balance can be achieved. A threshold of 30-45 Kcal/kg LBM/day is already considered low and athletes should only remain at this threshold for a short period of time. In any case, the studies reviewed by these authors showed that a threshold lower than 30 Kcal/kg BML/day seems to be the one at which serious health implications are found after only 5 days in healthy women.(22). Furthermore, they add that, after four days at a threshold between 19 and 25 kcal/kg, there was a reduction in triiodothyronine (T3) in exercising women who were previously inactive. Overall, chronic training induces a slight physiological increase in thyroid hormones in elite strength athletes and endurance runners, which may, to some extent, counteract the reduction in T3 and NEAT (non-exercise activity thermogenesis) [22].Taken together, these authors [22] suggest that as energy availability decreases, either intentionally through calorie restriction or involuntarily through increased exercise energy expenditure, metabolic adaptations will occur. Although these alterations are normal and insignificant if athletes return to an adequate energy intake, for example, after a structured diet phase, they can be problematic in individuals who have a constant drive to lose weight. While body weight will decrease at the beginning a diet phase, there will inevitably be a plateau in weight loss prolonged low energy intake. Although this a normal physiological adaptation, some athletes may begin to decrease energy intake even further in order to continue losing weight. This behaviour will lead to a downward spiral of calorie restriction, weight loss and plateau followed by another cycle, all of which will ultimately result in LEA [(22)]. They add that after a 5-day LEA, fasting blood glucose and insulin levels decrease, while β-hydroxybutyrate ketone (BHB) increases. In athletes with the triad, hypoglycaemia and hypercholesterolaemia are common. In contrast to the cardioprotective role of exercise, altered cholesterol levels may be unfavourable to cardiovascular health. The results of this review indicate that the reduction in glycolytic activity and increase in lipolytic activity during LEA occurs because of fuel sparing from carbohydrates. This is possibly due to limited glycogen stores. They add that fat stores in high-performance athletes are often close to the lower limit of 5% for men and 12% for women, especially in athletes involved in endurance or aesthetic sports [(22)].

Southmayd et al (2017), [(23)] in their study on nutritional treatment in relation to the pharmacological options of the female athlete triad, note that the first line of treatment to both restore menstrual function and improve bone health in women with FHA is to address energy deficiency by increasing food intake and reducing training load. They place particular importance on the concept of menstrual recovery which should include criteria such as: 3 consecutive cycles of less than 36 days, resumption of menstruation accompanied by a specific increase in oestrogen concentration during the follicular phase and ovulation or evident corpus luteum formation observed by increases in progesterone in the luteal phase. These criteria result in increased associations between menstrual recovery and bone health, as exposure to oestrogen is likely to be greater [(23)]. In this review [(23)], they target a weight gain of approximately 0.5 kg every 7 to 10 days by increasing energy intake by 20% to 30% above initial needs. According to these authors, there is no clear threshold of fat versus weight gain that determines menstrual or bone recovery. In any case, they understand that the benefits of weight regain on bone health are twofold: resumption of menstruation corrects hypoestrogenism to regulate low bone resorption and adequate energy reserves improve the hormonal profile to regulate bone formation. The most clinically important predictors of HPO axis recovery are weight gain and BMI. They add that a 2.7 kg increase in body weight in an amenorrheic athlete achieved by increasing energy intake by 360 Kcal/day restored LH pulsatility resembling the pattern observed in women. eumenorrhoeic women. In addition, they reported significant increases in body weight of about 5 kg (58.0 ± 2.0 to 63.3 ± 2.3 kg) in women who resumed menses, compared with non-significant increases in body weight of 1.3 kg (57.7 ± 3.2 to 59.0 ± 3.4 kg) in women who did not resume menses. In addition, they note that the odds of persistent amenorrhoea doubles for each 1 kg/m^2 reduction in BMI. These data highlight the important relationship between oestrogen status and energy status.

- **Calcium and vitamin D:**

Calcium and vitamin D are fundamental to the bone health of female athletes, as both nutrients play critical roles in the formation and maintenance of strong bones. Calcium contributes to bone density, reducing the risk of fractures and injuries, which are common in high-impact sports. Vitamin D, on the other hand, facilitates calcium absorption in the gut, ensuring that the mineral is available for proper bone mineralisation. In addition, both nutrients are essential for muscle function; calcium aids in muscle contraction and neuromuscular coordination, while vitamin D improves muscle strength and function. Deficiency of these nutrients can lead to bone weakness, increasing the risk of stress fractures and injury. According to this study (23), daily calcium intake recommendations are between 1000 and 1300 mg/day. In the case of vitamin D, in female long-distance runners, calcium supplementation of 800 mg/day, added to a usual dietary calcium intake of approximately 1000 mg/day, prevented BMD loss in the femur, compared to a 2% decrease in BMD in placebo-treated female runners. Calcium and vitamin D supplementation has also been shown to be beneficial in reducing the risk of developing stress fractures from strenuous training. They mention a study in female soldiers in which the intake of 2000 mg/day of calcium and 800 IU/day of vitamin D showed a 21% reduction in the incidence of stress fractures compared to those treated with placebo. In addition, they suggest that in energy-deficient female athletes, increased calcium and vitamin D intake may be the result of increased caloric intake (23).

- **Caloric intake considerations**

Adequate development of caloric intake in female athletes is crucial to optimise performance and overall health. An adequate caloric intake Adequate calorie intake provides the energy needed to support the intense training and physical demands of sport, helping to maintain endurance and athletic ability. If insufficient calories are consumed, it can result in fatigue, decreased performance and inadequate recovery after exercise. In addition, a prolonged calorie deficit can lead to loss of muscle mass and negatively affect bone health, increasing the risk of fractures and disorders such as amenorrhoea. Adequate caloric intake also ensures that the body has the nutrients necessary for essential metabolic functions, such as hormone regulation and cell repair.

Wohlgemuth et al (24), define energy availability (EA) as the energy remaining after taking into account the energy expenditure of physical activity; this energy is available for use in the body's vital metabolic processes. Five consecutive days (22,24) of low EA (< 30 kcal/kg LBM/day) in women resulted in a decrease in carbohydrate availability, which would have direct implications for performance. They aim for an optimal AE of 40-45 kcal/kg LBM/day to maintain bone health and maintain metabolism. In addition, it may be beneficial to increase caloric and certain macronutrient intakes throughout certain phases of the menstrual cycle (24).

- **Carbohydrates** (24)

Carbohydrates are a vital source of fuel during moderate to high intensity exercise. Currently, the acceptable macronutrient distribution range for carbohydrates is 45-65% of total calories with recommendations of 6-10 g/kg/day in active subjects. The requirements for this macronutrient are highly dependent on the duration and intensity of training, with longer and more intense activities increasing the demand.The correlation between performance and muscle glycogen content suggests that carbohydrate loading strategies may increase performance. Since most loading studies focus on men, it was assumed that similar guidelines would be applicable to women. However, this review notes that men and women differ in carbohydrate loading capacity following the same protocol. For example, they mention a study in which they applied a protocol that increased carbohydrate intake from 55% to 70% in male and female cyclists trained for 4 days. The women, who were in the follicular phase of the menstrual cycle, showed no significant changes in muscle glycogen content or performance. in a submaximal endurance test while men improved in both parameters (41% and 45% respectively). This is because, although the 4-day load was equal in both sexes, the absolute daily carbohydrate intake is higher in men, thus highlighting the importance of meeting the g/kg/day carbohydrate recommendations especially in women. These authors note, in their review, that a high carbohydrate diet (8.2 g/kg/day) results in a higher muscle glycogen content (13%) and better performance in a submaximal endurance test compared to a moderate carbohydrate diet (4.7 g/kg/day). They also conclude that women can perform carbohydrate loading during both phases of the menstrual cycle following the recommendations of 8-10 g/Kg/day in the 3 days prior to the event; however, with lower chronic intake, glycogen storage appears to be more effective with short-term carbohydrate increases in the luteal phase of the menstrual cycle when carbohydrate oxidation rates are high.

Regarding the effects of carbohydrate supplementation during prolonged endurance exercise, during the follicular and luteal phases, ingestion of a 6% carbohydrate solution every 15 minutes improves performance and minimises differences in blood glucose concentration between phases of the menstrual cycle. In addition, consumption of 500-1000 ml of the 6% carbohydrate solution is within the common guidelines for endurance athletes of 30-60 g/hour.After prolonged endurance exercise, the replenishment of muscle glycogen stores is a priority. In women, the ability to replenish stores fluctuates throughout the menstrual cycle, with the greatest capacity occurring during the follicular phase. In addition, this review includes that delayed carbohydrate intake in the immediate post-exercise period (2 hours) results in reduced rates of glycogen storage. Therefore, women should focus on the rapid consumption of at least 0.75 g/kg carbohydrate after prolonged exercise to restore glycogen consumed during exercise.In this review (24), they add the general recommendations for carbohydrate intake in female athletes as follows: In preparation for prolonged endurance exercise (> 90 minutes), women might consider carbohydrate loading by consuming 8-10 g/kg body weight in the 3 days prior to the event, especially if the event occurs in the follicular phase. In the hours leading up to the event, 1 g/kg body weight should be prioritised to ensure carbohydrate availability. during activity. During prolonged endurance exercise, women should consume 500-1000 ml of 6% carbohydrate solution per hour. After exercise, women should rapidly consume at least 0.75 g/kg of carbohydrate to begin the process of replenishing muscle glycogen stores.

• Fats (24)

Adequate fat intake is essential for female athletes for several key reasons. Fats, particularly healthy fats such as omega-3 and omega-6 fatty acids, play a crucial role in overall health and athletic performance. First, they provide a dense source of energy, crucial for maintaining endurance during long, intense workouts, as each gram of fat provides approximately 9 calories, compared to 4 calories per gram of protein and carbohydrates.Fats are also essential for the absorption of fat-soluble vitamins, such as vitamins A, D, E and K, which are essential for bone health, immune function and muscle recovery. In particular, vitamin D, found in some high-fat foods, is vital for bone health and hormone regulation. In addition, essential fatty acids, such as omega-3, have anti-inflammatory properties that can help reduce muscle soreness and inflammation, speeding post-workout recovery.Adequate fat intake is also crucial for hormone regulation, including sex hormones that affect reproductive function and the menstrual cycle. Insufficient fat intake can lead to hormonal imbalances and problems such as amenorrhoea, which can negatively affect health and performance. Finally, fats help maintain cellular integrity and cell membrane function, which is important for overall health and optimal performance.In this review, Wohlgemuth et al (24) note that fats are essential for the maintenance of sex hormone concentrations and for the absorption of fat-soluble vitamins. For women, adequate fat intake can help maintain normal menstrual cycles. Women should allocate 20% of total calories to fats, taking into account that there are additional recommendations for omega-6 (linoleic acid) and omega-3 (α-linoleic acid) fatty acids, which are recommended at 12 g and 1.1 g/day respectively in a ratio of 5-10:1. Finally, they should aim to obtain at least 15% of total calories from unprocessed fat sources. Furthermore, they add that variations in female sex hormones during the follicular and luteal phases of the menstrual cycle influence fat metabolism. Elevated oestrogen levels during the luteal phase promote lipolysis through increased sensitivity to lipoprotein lipase and increased growth . During the follicular phase, oestrogen levels are lower, resulting in less reliance on fat as an energy substrate. Therefore, there is a greater reliance on fat oxidation in the luteal phase versus the follicular phase. They conclude that more emphasis should be placed on dietary fat intake during the luteal phase of the menstrual cycle to support the increased reliance on fat metabolism.

•Proteins [24]

Muscle maintains a constant balance between muscle protein breakdown (MPB) and muscle protein synthesis (MPS). Maintaining adequate protein intake is paramount to ensure that the rate of MPS is at least equal to that of MPB to maintain muscle mass. The current recommended dietary allowance (RDA) for protein for all sedentary adults over the age of 18 years is 0.8 g/Kg/day. However, in this review they point out that the figure appears to be outdated and is based on a nitrogen balance method that may not be as accurate as recent techniques. It has also been suggested that it may be misinterpreted as an optimal level of protein intake rather than a minimum level to prevent muscle loss. In addition, they suggest that women are likely to need a higher protein intake due to increased protein oxidation; it has been suggested that the starting point for women is 1.6 g/kg/day, although more studies in women are needed to determine this.Female sex hormones (oestrogen and progesterone) peak during the mid-luteal phase, which corresponds to an increase in protein oxidation at rest. It is known that women need more lysine during the luteal phase than during the follicular phase for reasons related to the regulation of amino acid use by progesterone. The progesterone peak during the mid-luteal phase has been linked to a reduction in plasma amino acid levels as a result of increased biosynthesis. of protein due to the thickening of the endometrium. Increased protein intake during the mid-luteal phase is justified by the anabolic demands of the body especially when exercising. When combined with resistance training, increased protein intake has a synergistic effect with increased strength and muscle mass, i.e. hypertrophy. In the case of female athletes, this review notes that the average protein requirement is 1.63 g/kg/day during the follicular phase of the menstrual cycle. With the increased protein oxidation in the luteal phase, the needs will be increased. The phase of the cycle should be taken into account when assessing the dietary protein requirements of female athletes. In this review (24) they suggest that women have higher daily protein requirements than the current recommended amount of 0.8 g/kg/day. Strength and endurance athletes should consume at least 1.6 g/Kg/day. Spreading consumption throughout the day in 20-30 g servings is more optimal in relation to a larger intake or smaller, more frequent intakes.

4.13. Use of supplements in the female athlete

- **Beta-alanine (24)**

Beta-alanine is an important supplement for female athletes because of its significant impact on physical performance and endurance. This non-essential amino acid contributes to the synthesis of carnosine, a dipeptide that acts as an acid buffer in muscles. Carnosine helps neutralise the lactic acid that builds up during intense exercise, reducing muscle acidosis and fatigue. By decreasing lactic acid build-up, beta-alanine enables athletes to maintain a higher level of performance during prolonged, high-intensity activities. In addition, beta-alanine can improve training capacity and speed recovery between sessions. This is crucial for women who train intensively and are looking to maximise their results. Studies have shown that beta-alanine supplementation can increase exercise duration and improve performance in exercises lasting 1-4 minutes, such as sprinting and interval training. Wohlgemuth et al., (2021), state how this supplement is a non-essential amino acid that improves exercise performance increasing muscle carnosine levels and acts as a hydrogen ion buffer, thereby reducing pH. Increased muscle carnosine has been shown to result in improvements in exercise performance lasting mainly 2-4 minutes. Although most of the data on beta-alanine supplementation are from men, it has been found that, in women, initial muscle carnosine levels are lower, suggesting that they may derive greater benefits compared to men. In addition, carnosine levels are higher in women who consume more protein in their diet, and are therefore able to delay fatigue than women with lower carnosine levels. In relation to this supplementation, a slow-release supplement taken 6 g/day for 28 days will increase muscle carnosine levels by 16.4% more than taking a fast-release supplement. Beta-alanine supplementation recommendations should not differ between men and women. It is recommended to be taken at a total dose of 4-6 g/day divided into 1-2 g doses over the course of the day. In general, it can be effective in delaying fatigue and/or optimising recovery in women. It should be noted that it often produces a side effect of paraesthesia or tingling; and may be more common in men than in women.

- **Caffeine [(24)]**

Adequate caffeine intake is of great importance for female athletes due to its multiple benefits on sports performance and recovery. As a central nervous system stimulant, caffeine improves concentration and alertness, which is crucial for optimising quick decision-making during intense competition or training. This increase in concentration can help maintain accurate focus and execute sporting techniques more effectively.From a physical perspective, caffeine has a positive impact on endurance and exercise capacity. It increases the release of adrenaline, which prepares the body for intense exertion by mobilising fat for energy rather than primarily using carbohydrates. This effect is particularly beneficial for prolonged endurance events, where increased use of fat as an energy source can help conserve glycogen stores and delay fatigue [(24)]. In addition, caffeine reduces the perception of exertion, making exercise feel less strenuous. This may allow female athletes to train harder and longer before reaching exhaustion, thus improving performance capacity in training and competition. The ability to tolerate higher training volume and intensity can lead to significant improvements in overall performance and sporting results.

Caffeine also has positive effects on muscle strength and power. It increases the release of calcium into muscle cells, which optimises muscle contractions and can lead to improvements in strength and power during exercise. This is beneficial for sports that require explosiveness and strength, such as weightlifting and sprinting. It is important for female athletes to carefully manage their caffeine intake. The optimal dose may vary from person to person and it is essential to avoid excess, as it can cause adverse effects such as jitters, insomnia and gastrointestinal distress. Experimenting with the amount and timing of consumption is therefore essential to maximise benefits and minimise side effects. Caffeine is a natural ergogenic aid that elicits a physiological response by acting on adenosine receptors as a central nervous system stimulant. Caffeine elimination fluctuates throughout the menstrual cycle, with some women feeling the effects of caffeine longer in the luteal phase. This review shows that women may accumulate caffeine during the luteal phase before menstruation begins, and experience the effects caffeine for longer. In addition, these effects may increase premenstrual symptoms in some women, as well as intensify the normal effects of caffeine, i.e. increased heart rate, anxiety and sleep disturbance. They also add that caffeine (6 mg/kg) is effective for aerobic exercise performance, as it saves muscle glycogen by increasing fat metabolism. Caffeine is known to decrease pain perception, which would be useful before any type of exercise. Doses of between 3 and 9 mg/kg provide ergogenic effects when consumed 60 minutes before exercise (24).

- **Omega 3 (24)**

Omega-3 is a type of essential fatty acid that offers multiple benefits for female athletes, positively influencing their overall health and athletic performance. These fatty acids, especially EPA (eicosapentaenoic) and DHA (docosahexaenoic), found mainly in fatty fish and certain vegetable oils, are known for their anti-inflammatory properties and cardiovascular benefits.

In the context of sports, omega-3 plays a crucial role in reducing muscle inflammation. Intense training and competition can cause oxidative stress and inflammation in muscles, which in turn can cause soreness and delay recovery. Adequate omega-3 intake helps mitigate these effects by reducing the production of inflammatory molecules, thereby speeding muscle recovery and reducing the risk of injury. In addition, omega-3 improves cardiovascular health by lowering blood pressure and triglyceride levels. Good cardiovascular health is critical to athletic performance, as an efficient circulatory system ensures an adequate supply of oxygen and nutrients to muscles during exercise, which improves endurance and overall performance.DHA, in particular, is essential for brain health and cognitive function. For female athletes, optimal cognitive function is crucial for fast and effective decision-making during competitions and training. DHA helps maintain neuronal health and can improve focus, concentration and memory, key aspects of athletic performance.

Omega-3 also has a positive impact on body composition and metabolic regulation. It can help reduce body fat and increase lean muscle mass, which is beneficial for maintaining optimal body weight and improving performance in various sports disciplines. It is important for female athletes to incorporate an adequate amount of omega-3s into their diet to reap these benefits. Although omega-3s can be obtained from dietary sources such as oily fish, supplements may be a convenient option to ensure adequate intake, especially if fish consumption is limited. The Wohlgemuth et al. (2021) notes that omega-3 supplementation may help address the increased inflammatory response seen in women after exercise; increased omega-3 levels have also been shown to reduce symptoms of depression and anxiety, especially in women. women. In addition, they mention that to see the benefits of omega-3s, 1 to 3 g per day should be consumed [(24)].

•Probiotics [24]

This review highlights the benefits of probiotics for general health, highlighting their ability to improve the bacterial composition of the gut, regulate immune and digestive function, and support urogenital tract and skin health. A relevant aspect mentioned in the review is the positive impact of probiotics on nutrient absorption, particularly in improving iron levels. A recent study, focusing on women, showed that combining 20 mg of iron in the form of ferrous fumarate with the probiotic strain Lactobacillus plantarum resulted in improved iron absorption. This finding is crucial for women, who are at increased risk of developing iron deficiency anaemia due to the periodic blood loss associated with menstruation [24. Probiotics offer a potential solution to improve iron status, thus contributing to the reduction of the risk of anaemia. It is important to choose the right probiotics based on the specific strain and desired outcome, as needs may vary between women and men [(24)]. Taking a multi-strain probiotic supplement may be the best strategy for a full range of health benefits. To maximise these benefits, it is recommended that the probiotic supplement be taken daily and contain between 10 and 20 billion colony forming units (CFU), or include a clinically validated strain at effective doses. This will ensure that the desired effects on gut health and absorption of essential nutrients are achieved, thus supporting women's overall wellbeing and health.

•Protein supplements [24]

In relation to protein supplementation, this review adds that women could benefit from protein supplementation to meet their daily protein needs, especially during luteal phase of the menstrual cycle, which is characterised by increased protein oxidation. There are several types: essential amino acids, vegetable and whey proteins. Essential amino acids (EAA) are important for muscle protein synthesis and can have ergogenic effects. These authors mention that the literature has shown that six weeks of EAA supplementation (18.3 g/day) improves aerobic muscular endurance. In addition, consumption of 6-12 g of EAAs alone or as part of a 20-40 g protein supplement can stimulate protein synthesis. muscle protein. Plant-based proteins have also become popular sources of protein supplements and are usually from legumes, nuts or soya. Due to the amino acid profiles of the different plant sources, it is necessary to combine several types. If a plant-based protein is consumed, it is recommended that a probiotic be added as a way to enhance amino acid absorption. This technique ensures that enough leucine is consumed to stimulate MPS. Whey protein is the highest quality form of protein and is available as hydrolysate, isolate and concentrate. Whey protein isolate is pure, with a protein concentration of over 90%, as lactose and fat have been removed, and may be more beneficial for women to avoid gastrointestinal distress. Previous data have supported the use of protein before and/or after exercise in women to improve muscle recovery [(24)].

•Vitamins and minerals [(24)]

In relation to vitamins and minerals, these authors suggest that their use in the form of supplements may benefit very active people. Athletes who are menstruating may have a greater need for certain vitamins and minerals. In particular, female athletes are often deficient in folate, riboflavin and vitamin B12. Folate and B12 deficiencies can cause anaemia, which decreases athletic performance. The average intake of folates in women is 126-364 μg/day. This is well below the current RDA of 400 μg/day. Folate supplementation is a simple and effective method to meet current recommendations and avoid performance decline. The RDA for riboflavin is 1.1 mg/day for women. Riboflavin intake is usually 1.4 mg per 1000 calories, but women who are exercising or breastfeeding should consume 1.6 mg per 1000 calories. The RDA for B12 for adults is 2.4μg/day. People following plant-based diets are often deficient in

B12, as it is mainly consumed from meat and its bioavailability is low in vegetables. In addition to deficiency of B vitamins, some people also lack vitamin D. The RDA for vitamin D is 600 IU for men and women aged 9 to 70 years. The literature has shown that doses of 2000 to 4000 IU are safe and beneficial. In the case of decreased BMD, vitamin D plays an important role in promoting bone health. People with vitamin D deficiency may have poor bone mineralisation and suffer from bone problems, especially as they age. Women athletes have a lower calcium intake than men. In addition, those who are intolerant to dairy products are at even greater risk of calcium deficiency. The RDA for calcium for adult women is 1000 mg/day. Supplementation is a viable alternative for athletes who do not consume dairy or who have insufficient calorie intake. Calcium is also vital for muscle contraction and relaxation; therefore, supplementation can promote optimal muscle function. Iron deficiencies are very common among female athletes, especially those who are vegan/vegetarian and consume few calories. The ISSN recommends that men consume 8 mg/day, while women should consume 18 mg/day [(24).]

- **Creatine monohydrate [24, 25]**

Creatine works by increasing phosphocreatine stores in the muscles, resulting in increased energy availability during intense exercise. This increase in energy availability may improve athletic performance, especially in activities that require explosiveness and high intensity, such as weightlifting and sprinting. However, the current literature review [24] reveals a significant gap in research on creatine supplementation in women, especially during specific phases such as menstruation, pregnancy and postpartum. Although extensive studies have been conducted in men and athletes in general, the efficacy and safety of creatine in these stages of female life are not yet fully established. In addition, the review highlights that as women age, creatine may offer additional benefits beyond sports performance. It has been observed that creatine supplementation may contribute to improved general health and has potential positive effects on mental health, bone health and brain health. In particular, creatine may help mitigate the loss of muscle mass and bone density that often occurs with age, as well as support cognitive function and emotional stability. However, the evidence in these areas is still emerging and requires further research to confirm these benefits and to better understand how creatine supplementation can be safely and effectively integrated into women's lives throughout their lifespan [24].Smith-Ryan (2021) [(25)] suggest that women may experience an increase in muscle mass and function when they consume a dose of creatine for at least 7 consecutive days. Creatine supplementation alone or in combination with resistance training does not appear to provide benefits on bone physiology in postmenopausal women. However, when combined with resistance training, the vast majority of research supports the efficacy of supplementation in improving strength and physical performance in postmenopausal women [(25)]. Indeed, it may improve cognitive abilities, regulate mood and offer neuroprotection, especially in women. Although men appear to be more sensitive to creatine supplementation, improved athletic performance and increased fat-free mass have been observed in both sexes [(24)].

There are two effective strategies for increasing creatine stores in the body, each with its own characteristics and time of effect. The first strategy, known as the loading phase, involves ingesting 0.3 g of creatine per kilogram of body weight, divided into four daily doses, over a period of 5 to 7 days. This loading phase is designed to rapidly saturate the muscles with creatine. This is followed by a maintenance phase in which a daily dose of 3-5 grams is consumed to keep creatine levels in the muscles elevated. This strategy is effective in achieving a significant increase in creatine stores in a short period of time and can be beneficial for improving performance in activities that require explosiveness and high intensity.

The second strategy involves ingesting a constant daily dose of 5 grams of creatine, without a pre-loading phase. Although this strategy is less aggressive and may be easier to follow in the long term, it takes longer to build up muscle creatine stores to optimal levels. This option is suitable for those who prefer a more gradual approach, avoiding possible side effects related to the loading phase.Both strategies can provide the benefits associated with creatine supplementation, such as improvements in strength, power and muscle recovery. However, it is important to consider the potential side effects. A common side effect of creatine supplementation is weight gain, which is related to water retention in the muscles. This effect is more prevalent in men, but can also occur in women, especially during the luteal phase of the menstrual cycle due to hormonal changes that can influence fluid retention. It is crucial to note that the weight gain associated with the creatine can be transient and usually is related to muscle water content, not to an increase in fat mass. Therefore, although creatine supplementation may lead to weight gain in some cases, this effect is generally reversible and should not be a significant impediment to those seeking to improve their physical performance.

5. DISCUSSION

Throughout the development of this review, we seek to highlight that Functional Hypothalamic Amenorrhoea (FHA) should not be considered merely as an absence of menstruation, but as a complex disorder that requires a thorough understanding of the origin of the problem for its adequate solution. FHA is intrinsically linked to significant endocrine disturbances, which demonstrate that it is not just a deficit in menstruation, but a broader metabolic and hormonal imbalance. There is consensus that AHF is associated with a hypometabolic state, which is a consequence of a central inhibition of the reproductive axis. This imbalance is caused by the influence of stress hormones and endorphins, which interfere with the production and release of gonadotropin-releasing hormone (GnRH) in the hypothalamus. In turn, decreased levels of IGF-I (insulin-like growth factor 1) and leptin, hormones essential for energy homeostasis, contribute to this dysfunction. Leptin, in particular, plays a key role in regulating energy balance and the menstrual cycle. Low availability of these essential hormones results in reduced stimulation of the pituitary gland, which produces less luteinising hormone (LH) and follicle stimulating hormone (FSH). This reduction in hormone signalling prevents adequate oestrogen production in the ovaries, leading to anovulation and the absence of menstruation. As a result, the body enters a new adaptive metabolic state, in which the lack of regular hormonal signalling affects not only the menstrual cycle, but also general health and well-being. Therefore, addressing FHA requires an intervention that not only addresses the absence of menstruation, but also provides for the restoration of hormonal and metabolic balance for a full recovery.

Figure 5: Energy deficiency.

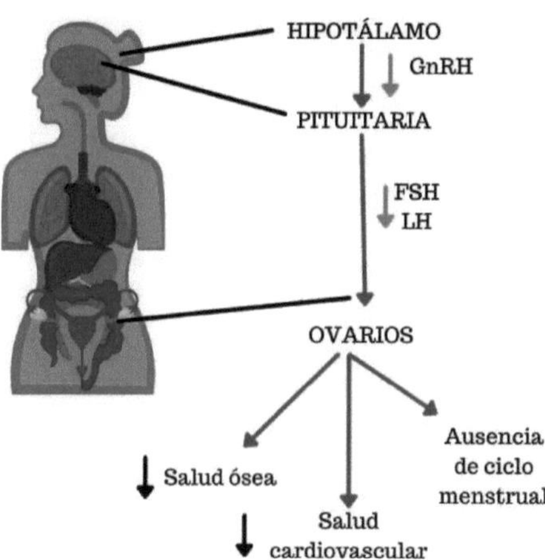

One of the main strengths of the present study is the assessment of metabolic, psychological and socio-cultural risk factors as possible contributors to the development of FHA. Particular emphasis has been placed on mental health (MH) with the intention of finding out whether they are a cause of RED-S, as although there are studies that suggest that young athletes experience similar mental health problems to non-athletes [(2)], it should be noted that they suffer from unique stressors that put them at risk of developing or exacerbating mental health disorders. Among the findings of the present review is that significantly more young female athletes with FHA also have a higher prevalence of subclinical dysfunctional eating behaviours [(3)]. The existing literature highlights the need for the development of questionnaires for the assessment of disordered eating behaviours and wellness education for young athletes, as well as the development of services that recognise the special needs of this population. The environment needs to be aware of the higher prevalence of disordered eating in these populations, as well as the diversity of symptoms. The present study provides significant information on the complex nature of FHA confirming the notion that FHA is a disorder. multidimensional and stresses that both metabolic and psychosocial factors are involved in the pathogenesis of the disorder. On the other hand, the results of this review highlight the complexity inherent in the diagnosis of Functional Hypothalamic Amenorrhoea (FHA), especially when associated with excessive exercise and relative energy deficit (RED). This complexity arises because many women with FHA are misdiagnosed with polycystic ovary syndrome (PCOS) due to the lack of a complete and thorough diagnostic work-up. Often, performing an ultrasound scan alone is not enough to make an accurate diagnosis of FHA, as affected women may have features that are also seen in PCOS, such as polycystic ovaries and certain symptoms of hyperandrogenism, such as facial hair. This overlapping of symptoms can lead to misdiagnosis and, consequently, inappropriate treatment. Thus, many women find themselves in the position of treating a pathology that does not correspond to their actual condition, which can lead to a lack of improvement in their symptoms and a possible prolongation of the underlying problem. In addition, there is a growing consensus that nutritional therapy and education should be the treatment of first choice for AHF associated with ALE. Correction of energy imbalance through proper diet and exercise management can restore menstrual and hormonal function more effectively than other interventions. On the other hand, the use of oral contraceptives (OCPs) as a treatment for AFH is considered suboptimal. Although OCPs may mask the symptom of absent menses, they do not address the underlying cause of the problem, which is hypothalamic-pituitary-ovarian (HPO) axis dysfunction. In fact, their prolonged use may make it difficult to normal endogenous hormone activity, further complicating the process of recovery and restoration of hormonal balance.The concept of energy availability, as well as its calculation, has evolved. In this review, we have tried to determine the limit value of this energy availability from which a multitude of alterations begin to occur in the organism, especially in the hypothalamic-pituitary-gonadal axis, in the hypothalamic-pituitary-thyroid axis and also in markers of bone formation and resorption in order to be able to apply appropriate nutritional strategies. Optimal energy availability in women is estimated to be above 45 Kcal/kg LBM/day and 30 Kcal/kg LBM/day is the LEA value which energy is no longer sufficient to maintain physiological functions. adequate. These values are not at all clear in athletes and there is some controversy; since many studies have been carried out in sedentary women, it should also be taken into account that the measurements carried out in laboratories, with highly controlled methods, differ greatly from reality, and are still poorly known in the case of men, possibly the field of LEA is the only one of sports nutrition that is more extensively studied in women than in men. The Female Athlete Triad is comprehensive concept that emerged to address and understand three interrelated and highly prevalent issues in female athletes: hypothalamic amenorrhoea (the absence of menstruation), eating disorders (ED) and osteoporosis. This initial concept, introduced to capture the complexity of these conditions, sought to connect how each might affect the overall health of female athletes and how they were interrelated. Hypothalamic amenorrhoea refers to the lack of menstruation due to hormonal dysfunctions associated with excessive exercise and energy deficit. Eating disorders, such as anorexia or bulimia, are often present in this context, exacerbating hormonal and nutritional problems. Osteoporosis, on the other hand, is a serious consequence of loss of bone mass due to inadequate diet and reduced bone mineral density. As research progressed, the concept of the Female Athlete Triad was refined to include Relative Energy Deficiency in Sport (READ) as a key causal factor. LEA refers to an imbalance between energy expenditure and caloric intake, which can occur both in the presence and absence of an eating disorder. This recognition expanded the original view of the triad, allowing for a better understanding of how energy insufficiency impacts the overall health of female athletes, affecting not only their menstrual cycle, but also their nutritional status and bone health.Over time, the concept of the triad was no longer seen as a fixed state but as a continuous pattern of change. This pattern represents a transition from a healthy to a pathological state, passing through various intermediate stages.

Rather than viewing the triad as a static set of conditions, it was understood that female athletes may experience different levels of severity and types of manifestations of these conditions over time.In order to address more inclusively other impairments that did not strictly fall under the triad and to apply the concept to an In a broader spectrum of athletes, including men, the term Relative Energy Deficiency in Sport was introduced. This concept encompasses a broader range of health impairments, not only endocrine and metabolic, but also psychological, haematological and immunological. ALE is recognised for its impact on health at multiple levels, affecting not only reproductive and bone function, but also general wellbeing and sporting performance. This includes consequences on mental health, the immune system and body composition, reflecting a more complete picture of how energy deficits affect athletes in general. The adoption of the term LEA provides a more holistic and adaptive view that allows for better identification and treatment of these conditions in diverse sporting populations.

Figure 6: Triad of the female athlete.

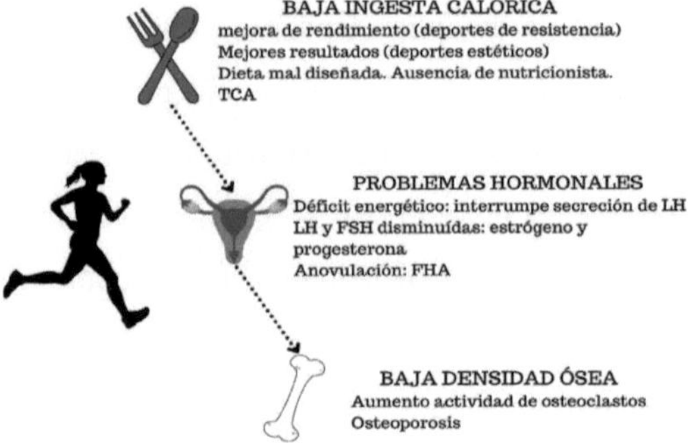

With regard to the knowledge of this pathology in the environment of sportswomen, this review highlights the need to raise awareness among professionals for its early detection, as it seems that they only have a partial knowledge of the symptoms. However, it is important to stress that the studies mentioned in this aspect are based on surveys that generate recruitment biases.

Even so, patient-centred and early detection studies are scarce. In this review, only two studies related to nutritional strategies and the use of sports supplementation to prevent this problem are mentioned, so this is the most important limitation of the study, as it was intended to answer the question of prevention. However, it does highlight that the focus is on energy and in particular the correct intake of carbohydrates. The new evidence underlines the importance of gender-specific nutritional strategies and recommendations, especially for active women.With regard to the decrease in BMD, through the analysis of the studies that deal with this problem, once again, this review highlights the need for early detection that would completely avoid the appearance of this problem. There are intra-individual differences in women, throughout the menstrual cycle and life cycle (puberty, pregnancy, menopause). These differences occur during the phases of the menstrual cycle, which are due to fluctuating hormone levels, for example, the increase in oestrogen and progesterone during the mid-luteal phase. Therefore, women can benefit from gender-specific nutritional recommendations, especially when they exercise regularly. Specific recommendations on calories, macronutrients, micronutrients and supplements should be tailored to each individual to achieve desired goals, but the basic requirements and starting points are likely to be universal and are therefore addressed in this review. In addition, timing and dosage should be considered, especially when performance or recovery are the primary goals. Such different nutritional guidelines and recommendations for women are warranted given the gender-based difference, but are lacking to date. There is also a significant lack of studies evaluating women's specific nutritional strategies for health, performance and body composition. More research evaluating women-specific nutritional strategies, especially for active women, is needed.It also highlights the desirability of multidisciplinary and individualised management of FHA cases, as well as the important role of the coach, teammates and social networks.

6. APPLICABILITY AND NEW LINES OF RESEARCH

The lack of clear and validated diagnostic methods in diverse populations is a major concern in the field of eating disorders and FHA (Functional Hypothalamic Amenorrhoea) research. It is essential to develop questionnaires that have been scientifically validated and to combine them with biochemical tests to obtain accurate diagnoses. In addition, monitoring of certain dietary behaviours can provide crucial information about these disorders. Accurate diagnosis will allow a better understanding of prevalence and associated risk factors, which is essential for designing effective interventions.

The need for future studies to elucidate the pathways by which psychosomatic factors contribute to the occurrence of disordered eating and FHA is evident. This review highlights the importance of a comprehensive assessment that includes not only gynaecological but also psychological aspects. Adolescent girls and young women with FHA often do not receive adequate psychological assessment, as both parents and health professionals focus on the gynaecological aspects of amenorrhoea. However, it is crucial to recognise that these women deserve a careful psychological evaluation to address all contributing factors to their condition.

For men, research on eating disorders and FHA is extremely limited. In addition, it is not known how long it will take for women affected by FHA to return to a normal menstrual cycle. Another area that requires more attention is the composition of the diet, beyond total energy intake. It is possible that the availability of certain macronutrients plays a crucial role, or perhaps it is the energy intake itself that determines the occurrence of all eating disorder (ED) disorders.Among athletes, the prevalence of ED is common, but there is still much to learn about how it varies within different sporting subgroups. While it has been clearly established that the emphasis on leanness is an important factor, the evidence in other subgroups is less conclusive. These findings are critical to guide future research seeking to define the prevalence of ED in various sports. Future research should focus on identifying pathological differences in the presentation of ED in various sporting categories. Specifically, patterns of ED in aesthetic and weight-dependent athletes should be addressed with special attention, as prevalence rates in these sports are particularly high. Screening tools developed to assess athletes should be validated across a wide range of athlete types, as the prevalence and manifestation of symptoms can vary significantly between different sports. Developing diagnostic tools or conducting research limited to a single population of athletes will greatly restrict the generalisability of results. Therefore, comprehensive and multi-sport research is needed, especially when dealing with athletes considered to be at high risk. Regarding the prevention of EDs, although numerous studies have been conducted on primary prevention, fewer studies have been conducted on early detection. This is a crucial issue, as early detection has been shown to significantly improve the prognosis of those affected. Improving knowledge levels among healthcare professionals is essential. This can be achieved through initial and continuing education programmes, such as e-learning, which is a cost-effective and efficient method of developing knowledge and skills.

E-learning programmes can reach a wide audience at relatively low cost, allowing effective distribution of educational materials. It is essential that this training is not limited to physicians and nutritionists, but includes any professional who can detect EDs early, such as endocrinologists and pharmacists. A critical area for early detection is the school environment, as school age is the most common period for the onset of eating disorders.

To improve early detection in schools, it is proposed to train school staff to identify students at risk of EDs, how to approach them appropriately and where to refer them care. Future research should focus on identifying methods to reduce barriers to help-seeking, such as stigma, shame, denial, lack of knowledge about EDs and negative attitudes towards treatment. Addressing these barriers may make it easier for more people to seek and receive appropriate treatment early, thereby improving their long-term outcomes.

7. CONCLUSIONS

Loss of menses in female athletes is a clear indicator that something is going on in the body that needs to be taken seriously, and should never be considered a normal part of training or sport. AHF is a manifestation of a state of low energy availability, which implies that the body is experiencing a deficit between caloric intake and energy expenditure. This deficit forces the body to implement a series of metabolic and physiological adaptations to reduce energy , additional weight loss and preserve survival under stressful conditions. In response to this energy-deficient state, the hypothalamus initiates an adaptive response that includes a reduction in GnRH secretion.

This decrease in GnRH directly affects the function of the pituitary gland, which produces lower amounts of LH and FSH. The reduction in LH and FSH levels causes a decrease in ovarian oestrogen production, leading to a state of hypoestrogenism. The lack of oestrogen prevents ovulation, resulting in functional hypothalamic amenorrhoea.If this condition persists over time, it can have serious consequences for women's health, especially bone health. Reduced oestrogen production contributes to an accelerated loss of bone mass, which increases the risk of developing osteoporosis and fractures. Compromised bone health can have a lasting impact on quality of life, reducing bone density and making bones more fragile and susceptible to injury. Although historically it was thought that exercise intensity alone might be the main cause of FHA, recent research has shown that the problem lies not only in the intensity of exercise, but in the lack of sufficient nutrient and energy intake needed to support that physical activity. This situation is known as Relative Energy Deficiency in Sport (RED-S). In this context, the critical factor is adequate energy intake. Energy deficiency in athletes can be the result of several factors, including disordered eating, disordered eating habits, TCA, intentional weight loss without the presence of psychological problems but with a poorly designed dietary plan, or simply insufficient nutrition without awareness of the magnitude of the energy deficit. The consensus in the scientific community is that the first line of treatment for AHF should be a nutritional intervention rather than a pharmacological intervention. Restoration of adequate energy intake is essential to restore hormonal balance and re-establish the menstrual cycle. However, despite this consensus, the current review has failed to establish specific and universal guidelines for the prevention and treatment of AIH. This is largely because each athlete has unique individual characteristics that require personalised intervention. Each case of ALF may involve different degrees of energy deficiency and nutritional needs, which means that intervention must be tailored to each person's particular situation. In addition, further research is needed to identify other nutritional factors that could influence the prevention and treatment of ALF beyond simply correcting energy intake. The lack of generalisable guidelines for the general athletic population indicates that there is still much to be discovered about how to optimise nutrition to effectively prevent and treat HAB. Future research should address these additional factors and develop strategies that are applicable to a wide range of athletes, taking into account individual variations and the different contexts in which energy deficiency occurs. In this way, more accurate and effective recommendations for maintaining reproductive and general health in female athletes can be provided.

8. BIBLIOGRAPHY

1. Sophie Gibson M.E., Fleming N., Zuijdwijk C. and Dumont T.Where Have the Periods Gone? The Evaluation and Management of Functional Hypothalamic Amenorrhea. J Clin Res Pediatr Endocrinol. 2020 Feb; 12 (Suppl 1): 18-27.

2. Xanthopoulos M.S., Benton T., Lewis J., Case J.A. and Master C.L.Mental Health in the Young Athlete.Curr Psychiatry Rep. 2020 Sep; 22 (11): 63.

3. Tranoulis A., Soldatou A., Georgiou D., Mavrogianni D., Loutradis D. and Michala L.Adolescents and young women with functional hypothalamic amenorrhoea: is it time to move beyond the hormonal profile?. Arch Gynecol Obstet. 2020 Apr; 301 (4): 1095-1101.

4. Mancine R.P., Gusfa D.W., Moshrefi A. and Kennedy S.F.Prevalence of disordered eating in athletes categorized by emphasis on leanness and activity type - a systematic review.J Eat Disord. 2020; 8: 47.

5. Petisco-Rodríguez C., Sánchez-Sánchez L.C., Fernández-García R., Sánchez-Sánchez J. and García-Montes J.M.Disordered Eating Attitudes, Anxiety, Self-Esteem and Perfectionism in Young Athletes and Non-Athletes. IJERPH. 2020 Sep; 17 (18): 6754.

6. Nina K., France H., Anne-Claire S., Caroline H. and Nathalie G.Early detection of eating disorders: a scoping review. EatWeight Disord. 2021 Mar; : 1-48.

7. Hirschberg A.L.Female hyperandrogenism and elite sport.Endocr Connect. 2020 Mar; 9 (4): R81-R92.

8. Anna K. Melin, Christian Ritz, Jens Faber, Jens Faber, Sven Skouby, et al. Impact of Menstrual Function on Hormonal Response to Repeated Bouts of

Intense Exercise. Front Physiol. 2019 Jul; 10: 942.

9. Lombardi G., Ziemann E., Banfi G. and Corbetta S.Physical Activity-Dependent Regulation of Parathyroid Hormone and Calcium-Phosphorous Metabolism.Int J Mol Sci. 2020 Jul; 21 (15).

10. Elliott-Sale K.J., McNulty K.L., Ansdell P., Goodall S., Hicks K.M., Thomas K., et al. The Effects of Oral Contraceptives on Exercise Performance in Women: A Systematic Review and Meta-analysis.Sports Med. 2020 Oct; 50 (10): 1785-1812.

11. Dhair A., Abed Y. and Spradley F.T.The association of types, intensities and frequencies of physical activity with primary infertility among females in Gaza Strip, Palestine: A case-control study.PLoS One. 2020; 15 (10): e0241043.

12. Heather A.K., Thorpe H., Ogilvie M., Sims S.T., Beable S., Milsom S., et al. Biological and Socio-Cultural Factors Have the Potential to Influence the Health and Performance of Elite Female Athletes: A Cross Sectional Survey of 219 Elite Female Athletes in Aotearoa New Zealand. Front Sports Act Living. 2021 Feb; 3: 601420.

13. Yeager K.K., Agostini R., Nattiv A. and Drinkwater B.The female athlete triad: disordered eating, amenorrhea, osteoporosis.Med Sci Sports Exerc. 1993 Jul; 25 (7): 775-7.

14. Committee Opinion No.702: Female Athlete Triad.Obstet Gynecol. 2017 Jun; 129 (6): e160-e167.

15. Williams N.I., Koltun K.J., Strock N.C.A. and De Souza M.J.Female Athlete Triad and Relative Energy Deficiency in Sport: A Focus on Scientific Rigor.Exerc Sport Sci Rev. 2019 Oct; 47 (4): 197-205.

16. De Souza M.J., Koltun K.J., Etter C.V. and Southmayd E.A.Current Status of the Female Athlete Triad: Update and Future Directions. Curr Osteoporos

Rep. 2017 Dec; 15 (6): 577-587.

17. David R. Hooper, Jared Mallard, Jeff T. Wight, Kara L. Conway, George G.A. Pujalte, Kelsey M. Pontius, et al. Performance and Health Decrements Associated With Relative Energy Deficiency in Sport for Division I Women Athletes During a Collegiate Cross-Country Season: A Case Series.Front Endocrinol (Lausanne). 2021; 12: 524762.

18. Moskvicheva Y.B., Gusev D.V., Tabeeva G.I. and Chernukha G.E. [Evaluation of nutrition, body composition and features of dietetic counseling for patients with functional hypothalamic amenorrhea].Vopr Pitan. 2018; 87 (1): 85-91.

19. Southmayd E., Mallinson R., Williams N. and De Souza M.J. Unique Effects of Energy versus Estrogen Deficiency on Components of Bone Strength in Exercising Women: 1801 Board #3 June 2, 1.
Science in Sports & Exercise. 2016 May; 48: 490-491.

20. Papageorgiou M., Dolan E., Elliott-Sale K.J. and Sale C.Reduced energy availability: implications for bone health in physically active populations. Eur J Nutr. 2018 Apr; 57 (3): 847-859.

21. Ogwumike, Omoyemi O. and Uba, Misbahu. Association Between Menstrual Cycle Status and Musculoskeletal Disorders Among Female Athletes in Nigeria. Journal of Women's Health Physical Therapy. 2018 Sep; 42 (3): 148-153.

22. Wasserfurth P., Palmowski J., Hahn A. and Kruger K.Reasons for and Consequences of Low Energy Availability in Female and Male Athletes: Social Environment,Adaptations,and Prevention.SportsMed Open. 2020 Sep; 6 (1): 44.

23. Southmayd E.A., Hellmers A.C. and De Souza M.J.Food Versus Pharmacy: Assessment of Nutritional and Pharmacological Strategies to Improve Bone

Health in Energy-Deficient Exercising Women. Curr Osteoporos Rep. 2017 Oct; 15 (5): 459-472.
24. Wohlgemuth K.J., Arieta L.R., Brewer G.J., Hoselton A.L., Gould L.M. and Smith-Ryan A.E.Sex differences and considerations for female specific nutritional strategies: a narrative review. J Int Soc Sports Nutr. 2021 Apr; 18 (1): 1-20.

25. Smith-Ryan A.E., Cabre H.E., Eckerson J.M., Candow D.G. and Diel P.Creatine Supplementation in Women's Health: A Lifespan erspective.Nutrients. 2021 Mar; 13 (3): 877-1.

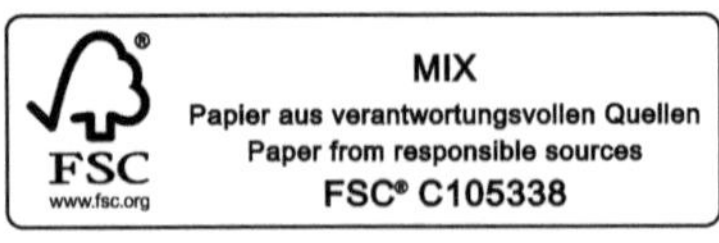

Printed by Books on Demand GmbH, Norderstedt / Germany